Natural Treatment Solutions For
Hyperthyroidism and Graves' Disease

Discover How Taking A Natural Thyroid Treatment Approach Can Restore Your Health... And Help You To Avoid Radioactive Iodine

Revised Third Edition

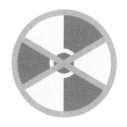

Eric M. Osansky, DC, MS, IFMCP

Natural Treatment Solutions for Hyperthyroidism and Graves' Disease
By Eric M. Osansky, DC, MS, IFMCP

Printed in the United States of America

Natural Endocrine Solutions
10020 Monroe Rd. Ste #170-280
Matthews, NC 28105

www.naturalendocrinesolutions.com
www.savemythyroid.com

Book design: Adina Cucicov

ISBN: 978-1-66640-408-1

A Word Of Caution To The Reader

This book is for educational purposes only, and is not intended to diagnose or treat any disease. Please do not apply any of this information without first speaking with your doctor. The content in this book is not intended to be a substitute for professional medical advice, diagnosis, or treatment. Always seek the advice of your physician or another qualified healthcare provider with any questions you may have regarding your health condition. You should also speak with your physician or other healthcare professional before taking any medication or nutritional, herbal or homeopathic supplements, or adopting any treatment for a health condition.

Video Summary

Do you want a video summary of this book that will help you to begin making progress on saving your thyroid?

Check out this free video training and overview of the process of reversing your hyperthyroidism and regaining your health

In this free training I cover 3 topics:

- Topic #1: Conventional vs. Natural Treatment Options for Hyperthyroidism
- Topic #2: Common thyroid healing roadblocks
- Topic #3: Important tips for those recently diagnosed with hyperthyroidism who are trying to avoid radioactive iodine and thyroid surgery

savemythyroid.com/video

○ v ○

Thyroid-Related Resources

I've included all of the references and many of the resources related to this book on the website listed below, although I did list some resources in Chapter 32. For those wondering why I didn't include most of the resources in this book, in the second edition of my book I did include specific resources, but since then some of the companies have gone out of business, while with others I just simply changed to a different option. There is almost no doubt that until I write a fourth edition of this book some of the resources I use and recommend will change, and it will be a lot easier to make changes to the resources listed on a website than it is to update this book.

To access the references and resources visit
savemythyroid.com/hyperbooknotes

Dedication

I dedicate this book to people with hyperthyroidism who are looking to do everything possible to preserve the health of their thyroid gland, and therefore avoid radioactive iodine and thyroid surgery.

Acknowledgements

First of all, I'd like to thank my wonderful wife Cindy for her continued love and support while writing this book.

Second, I'd like to commend all of the people with hyperthyroid conditions who are open minded enough to look for a natural treatment solution.

Third, I'd like to commend all of the other natural healthcare professionals who help find and remove their patient's triggers and underlying imbalances.

A SPECIAL INVITATION
The Hyperthyroid Healing COMMUNITY

In 2021 I started my "Hyperthyroid Healing" community, which currently consists of over 10,000 members. I wanted to create an online community where everyone with hyperthyroidism who is looking to save their thyroid can connect with others, ask questions, support one another, discuss the content in my book and podcast, swap recipes, etc.

You can immediately begin connecting with 10,000+ like-minded people with hyperthyroidism. Simply visit savemythyroid.com/community, and request to join the Hyperthyroid Healing Community (Facebook group). It's free to join, and while you'll find many people who are beginning their hyperthyroid healing journey, you'll also find others who were diagnosed with hyperthyroidism months or years ago, and who will happily share advice, support, and guidance, which in turn can help save your thyroid. In addition to trying to welcome all new members into the group, I try to do live Q & As in the group at least once or twice each month to answer questions.

By the way, I realize not everyone is on Facebook, and for different reasons some people prefer not to be on Facebook, which I completely understand. I can't say that I love Facebook, but I've tried different groups and the engagement just isn't the same.

Anyway, for those who are interested in joining I look forward to seeing you in the group!

Best of health,
Dr. Eric

Table of Contents

Introduction: Why a Natural Treatment Approach?..1

Chapter 1: What This Book Isn't About..11

Chapter 2: My Personal Story..21

Chapter 3: Hyperthyroidism vs. Graves' Disease: What's The Difference?...........29

Chapter 4: Finding The Underlying Cause Of Your Condition..............................35

Chapter 5: My True Feelings About Conventional Medical Treatment Methods....45

Chapter 6: Do Natural Treatment Methods Provide A Permanent Cure?..............53

Chapter 7: The Immune System Component Of Graves' Disease..........................63

Chapter 8: The Role That Stress Plays In The Development Of Hyperthyroidism....71

Chapter 9: The Importance Of Proper Digestion In Restoring Your Health...........89

Chapter 10: The Immune-Gut Connection And Graves' Disease...........................99

Chapter 11: Hyperthyroid Diet Tips...111

Chapter 12: Nutritional Supplements & Herbs For Hyperthyroidism & Graves' Disease..131

Chapter 13: The Truth About Iodine And Hyperthyroidism................................151

Chapter 14: Can Environmental Toxins Trigger Graves' Disease?.......................163

Chapter 15: The Role Of Infections In The Development Of Graves' Disease......181

Chapter 16: How Big Of A Role Does Genetics Play?..193

Chapter 17: Graves' Disease & Thyroid Antibodies...199

Chapter 18: 5 Reasons To Avoid Radioactive Iodine Treatment.........................209

Chapter 19: The Risks Of Playing The Waiting Game..223

Chapter 20: Combining Natural Treatment Methods With Conventional
Treatment Methods...231

Chapter 21: Can Thyroid Nodules Be Treated Naturally?.......................239

Chapter 22: Overcoming Thyroid Eye Disease..................................253

Chapter 23: Natural Treatment Methods During Pregnancy & Lactation..........267

Chapter 24: Can a Natural Treatment Approach Help With a Thyroid Storm?.....277

Chapter 25: Overcoming Toxic Multinodular Goiter...........................283

Chapter 26: 5 Reasons Why You Shouldn't Self-Treat Your Hyperthyroid Condition...291

Chapter 27: Natural Treatment Methods Don't Cure Anything..................297

Chapter 28: What Can You Do If Natural Treatment Methods Aren't Effective?...303

Chapter 29: The Keys To Maintaining Your Health............................317

Chapter 30: Consult With A Natural Healthcare Practitioner.................327

Chapter 31: Formulate An Action Plan To Restore Your Health................337

Chapter 32: Additional Natural Thyroid Health Resources....................343

Chapter 33: Twenty Three Questions You May Have...........................347

Thank you for reading my book!..363

Want to work with my team and I?..365

About The Author..367

Index...369

Why a Natural Treatment Approach?

MANY PEOPLE WHO have hyperthyroidism might wonder why they should consider taking a natural treatment approach. After all, if their endocrinologist or general medical practitioner has recommended anti-thyroid drugs or radioactive iodine treatment, then why question these conventional treatment methods? Since these doctors have been trained to help people with thyroid conditions it might seem to be foolish to attempt treating such a condition naturally.

Plus, most endocrinologists label hyperthyroidism and Graves' Disease as being incurable. Let's not forget we're talking about specialists who have received many years of training. So shouldn't they know better than some "wacky" holistic practitioner who claims that someone with a hyperthyroid condition can have their health restored through a natural treatment approach?

While it might make complete sense to follow the advice of your medical doctor without considering alternative treatment methods, one needs to keep a few things in mind. First of all, the reason why most endocrinologists advise their patients with hyperthyroidism and Graves' disease to take prescription drugs or receive radioactive iodine treatment is because this is how they have been trained. As you might have guessed, there is no functional medicine training in most medical schools, as doctors are taught to treat most conditions through drugs, surgery, and other conventional methods. And the same concept applies with the endocrinologist specialty, as they go through extensive training to obtain these credentials, but they are taught to treat most hyperthyroid conditions with antithyroid medication, radioactive iodine, or thyroid surgery.

While working towards getting my Master's degree in nutrition, one of the instructors held degrees in chiropractic and naturopathy, and he also graduated from osteopathic school. An osteopath's training is almost identical to those of medical doctors, as upon graduating they can diagnose, prescribe drugs, etc. In any case, he had graduated from one of the top colleges in the country, and I recall him talking about how nothing was taught to him about nutrition. And this is the case with most medical schools, as those attending such schools are not trained to address chronic conditions through diet, lifestyle, and environmental factors.

The Difference Between Medical Doctors, Chiropractors, and Naturopaths

There are numerous differences between the medical profession, and "alternative" healthcare practitioners such as chiropractors and naturopaths. While some medical doctors choose to learn more about functional medicine after graduating from medical school, most continue to do what they were taught in medical school. And in most cases they have been trained to diagnosis conditions, and then to manage the person's symptoms through medication, surgery, and other conventional procedures. Medical doctors are also trained to handle emergency procedures, and usually do a great job in this area.

The problem is that most medical doctors don't do anything to detect or address the underlying cause of the condition. For example, if a medical doctor has a patient with digestive problems, they will usually do one of two things. Depending on the problem they might recommend medication to manage the digestive symptoms. So if the person has acid reflux, they'll most likely recommend acid blocking medication, which just covers up the problem and most likely will make things worse. In some cases they might run a few tests, but if these come out negative they will usually tell the patient to live with the discomfort, or once again, may resort to medication for symptom management.

If someone is experiencing fatigue they might run a few tests, as they might run an iron panel and test the vitamin B12 levels, or perhaps run some different tests. Assuming these are negative then in most cases they will tell the patient there's nothing they can do, or perhaps they will recommend medication for symptom management. I've had many patients get turned away from their endocrinologists when they asked them to evaluate their adrenals. And when endocrinologists do evaluate the adrenals, most will only do a one sample cortisol test.

And of course the same concept applies with hyperthyroidism. Most medical doctors won't do anything to look into the cause of the condition. And if you tell them you're working with a natural healthcare professional, most won't be too supportive of this, and some endocrinologists might even refuse to continue treating your condition if you tell them you're taking a natural treatment approach.

On the other hand, chiropractors and naturopaths are taught to look for the underlying cause of the condition. While most chiropractors are associated with helping people who have neck and back pain conditions, the philosophy of chiropractic actually focuses on balancing the nervous system, as the nervous system controls every cell and tissue in the body. They do this through spinal adjustments, and although I think it's safe to say that most thyroid and autoimmune thyroid conditions aren't caused by spinal subluxations, I just wanted to briefly familiarize you with the chiropractic philosophy. Some chiropractors also incorporate nutrition and herbology into their practice. Naturopathic doctors also look into the cause of the condition, rather than just manage the symptoms.

Of course there are times when conventional medical treatment is necessary. So I'm not suggesting that everyone with Graves' disease or other types of hyperthyroidism shouldn't take antithyroid drugs, beta blockers, or receive thyroid surgery. Without question some people with hyperthyroid conditions do need to take medication to manage the symptoms, and some also will need to get thyroid surgery. But the reason why I wrote this book is because while some people do need to receive conventional medical treatment, many people with hyperthyroidism can restore their health through natural treatment methods. And many people who can't completely regain their health can still benefit from taking a natural treatment approach.

There Is No Official "Hyperthyroid Specialist"

While it's safe to say that many endocrinologists see a fair share of people with hyperthyroidism and Graves' disease, they also focus on other health conditions as well. This includes hypothyroidism and Hashimoto's thyroiditis, diabetes, and numerous other conditions. This isn't to suggest that these doctors aren't competent with hyperthyroidism, but my point is that they have to deal with other health conditions, and as a result most don't have the time to look into holistic methods to help their patients. And to be frank, most of these doctors probably don't have the desire to use natural treatment methods on their patients.

Once again, these doctors simply aren't trained in medical school to treat any health condition naturally. So when someone comes into their office with hyperthyroidism, or any other health condition, they don't think to themselves, "what is the actual cause of this condition?" Instead, they will run their set of tests, and then based on the test results they will put the person on the necessary medical protocol.

For diabetes, this frequently involves telling the person they will need to take insulin, or perhaps metformin daily for the rest of their life, although they will also need to inform the person of modifying what they can eat and drink. For hypothyroidism, they will almost always recommend for the patient to take synthetic thyroid hormone, rather than trying to find out why the person became hypothyroid to begin with (yes, natural treatment methods can benefit many of these people too!).

And with hyperthyroidism and Graves' disease, they will either have the patient take prescription drugs to manage the symptoms and possibly put the condition into a state of remission, which doesn't always happen, but when it does this is usually temporary. Or they will right off the bat advise the patient to receive radioactive iodine (RAI) treatment.

Why Not Find The Underlying Cause Of The Condition?

On the other hand, many natural healthcare practitioners take the opposite approach. While they might order the same thyroid blood tests and recommend other similar tests, a good natural healthcare practitioner will also try to determine the cause of the condition. Because by looking into the cause of the condition, many people with hyperthyroidism can restore their health by addressing that cause. And as I have already mentioned, for those people who can't have their health restored back to normal, many can still receive some great benefits from natural treatment methods, and at the very least prevent their condition from worsening over time.

For example, it is agreed by numerous healthcare practitioners that stress is a potential cause of hyperthyroidism and Graves' disease. And while there is no definitive way to determine whether stress has caused someone's condition, one can get a good idea of whether stress is a factor by looking at the patient's history, and also by evaluating the health of the patient's adrenal glands, which is almost never done by most medical doctors. And as I mentioned before, when they do recommend a test to determine the health of the adrenal glands, it is almost always a one-sample blood test of the morning cortisol levels, which in most cases isn't sufficient to get a complete picture of the health of the adrenals. Plus the stress of receiving the injection when doing the blood draw can falsely elevate the cortisol levels.

In any case, if it was determined that stress was a probable cause of someone's hyperthyroid condition, or at least a contributing factor, then one can help the patient to better cope with the stress in their life. Doing this alone probably wouldn't cure their hyperthyroid condition, but without question it is an important factor in restoring someone's health. And of course helping them cope with stress better can also prevent their condition from becoming worse over time.

The United States vs. Other Countries

Although I do have patients who live overseas, most of the people I work with live in the United States. And when compared to other countries, many medical doctors in the United States use invasive procedures on a more frequent basis. I'm not just talking about hyperthyroid conditions, but many other conditions as well. This would be fine if it led to a better outcome when compared to other countries, but this usually isn't the case.

For example, the most common surgery in the United States is the Caesarean section, which no doubt can save lives in many pregnant women. But the C-Section rate is much higher when compared to some other countries that have a much lower mortality rate. In other words, while some C-sections are without question necessary, many are done unnecessarily.

In fact, according to an article written in the New York Times, "The Caesarean section rate in the United States reached 32 percent in 2007, the country's highest rate ever".[1] A rate of around 15 percent would be ideal according to The World Health Organization. The article also states, "When needed, a Caesarean can save the mother and her child from injury or death, but most experts doubt that one in three women need surgery to give birth. Critics say the operation is being performed too often, needlessly exposing women and babies to the risks of major surgery."[2]

The same concept applies with the hysterectomy, as while this type of surgery is also necessary in some women, in many women this procedure is performed unnecessarily. Over 500,000 women receive this procedure each year. Don't get me wrong, as in the case of uterine cancer or other serious health issues, a hysterectomy may be warranted. But just as is the case with C-sections, many women receive a hysterectomy when there are alternative options.

According to Elizabeth Plourde, author of the book "Your Guide to Hysterectomy, Ovary Removal, & Hormone Replacement", "Though the first hysterectomies were implemented to save women's lives, now only 10% are the result of cancer, and less than 1% for obstetrical emergencies. The other, approximately 89%, are classified as "elective" surgery, and are performed for conditions that are not life-threatening.[3]

It's a similar situation with the thyroid gland, as many endocrinologists in the United States recommend radioactive iodine as the first line of treatment, whereas in many European countries, as well as other areas outside of the United States, radioactive iodine (RAI) isn't the preferred treatment method. In fact, one study looked at the differences in the diagnosis and treatment of Graves' disease in Europe, Japan, and the United States, and revealed that RAI was the treatment method of choice for 69% of doctors in the United States, but only 22% of European doctors recommended RAI as a first line of treatment, and only 11% of medical doctors in Japan recommended RAI as an initial treatment method.[4]

And while before I spoke about how medical doctors in the Unites States are more aggressive when it comes to recommending hysterectomies, one can argue that the thyroid gland is much more important than the uterus, or any other gland or organ frequently removed (gallbladder, appendix, etc.). While one can live without a uterus, gallbladder, tonsils, appendix, etc., nobody can live without a thyroid gland unless if they take synthetic or natural thyroid hormone. And the reason for this is because thyroid hormone supplies just about every tissue and cell in the body. So while nobody wants to have any gland or organ removed, one can argue that the thyroid gland is one of the last parts of the body you would want removed.

Try To Keep An Open Mind

In order to benefit from this book, it is important for you to keep an open mind. I of course don't expect you to agree with everything I say. In fact, I expect you to be skeptical. Just keep in mind that my goal isn't to convince you to take a natural treatment approach and avoid conventional medical treatment protocols. Instead, my goal is to show you the benefits of natural treatment methods, including how such treatment methods helped with my autoimmune hyperthyroid condition, along with many of the patients I have consulted with over the years who also had these conditions, and at the same time discuss the different benefits and risks of all of the different treatment options out there.

While I'm obviously biased towards natural treatment methods, I once again do realize that there is a time and place for conventional medical treatment, and I ultimately want to provide you with the information you need to make an informed decision. If after reading this book you choose to take a natural treatment approach then that's great. On the other hand, if you decide that conventional medical treatment methods are the best option for you, then that's fine too. Some people combine natural treatment methods with conventional medical treatment. Either way, as long as you have explored all of your options and feel comfortable with your decision, then I'll feel as if I did my job.

CHAPTER 1

What This Book Isn't About

THERE ARE A FEW different books out there related to hyperthyroidism and Graves' disease. Some of them go into great detail about the condition itself, giving a detailed explanation about how the thyroid gland works, the physiology of the endocrine system, the difference between T4 and T3, the different types of thyroid antibodies, etc. This book won't go into much detail with regards to the anatomy and physiology of the endocrine system, and it also won't give a detailed breakdown of the different thyroid blood tests, thyroid antibodies, etc.

If you want to know about the anatomy of the thyroid gland, receive a detailed breakdown of the different thyroid blood tests available, and to better understand the physiology, then there are a few different resources you can check out.

First of all, you might want to check out one or both of the following two books:

Book #1: *Graves' Disease: A Practical Guide* by Elaine A. Moore and Lisa Moore

Book #2: *Living Well with Graves' Disease and Hyperthyroidism: What Your Doctor Doesn't Tell You... That You Need To Know* by Mary J. Shomon

While there are other resources on hyperthyroidism and Graves' disease, both Mary Shomon and Elaine Moore have put together wonderful, well-researched books which focus on these conditions. In fact, if you were recently diagnosed with hyperthyroidism then you might even want to read these books before you read my book. Not that they're prerequisites, as my book is basic enough for most people to understand.

But for some people it's helpful to fully understand the basic anatomy and physiology as it pertains to hyperthyroidism and Graves' disease, gain a greater knowledge of the different thyroid blood tests, etc, before trying to understand why natural treatment methods are so effective. Just to let you know, while I think these both are great books, this doesn't mean I agree with everything these authors discuss. There are some things I disagree with, which is perfectly fine, as I'm sure there are some topics I discuss in this book which they will disagree with as well.

Another option is to check out my free Foundations of Overcoming Hyperthyroidism Online Course. This includes video lessons where I discuss some of the basics of overcoming hyperthyroidism. This definitely will benefit anyone who has recently been diagnosed with hyperthyroidism, but even if you've been dealing with hyperthyroidism for many years I'm confident that you will find the online course to be extremely valuable in your road to recovery. You can learn more about the online course by visiting savemythyroid.com/foundations.

What You Should Expect From Reading This Book

As I just mentioned, I try to keep this book very basic and easy to understand, as I don't go into great detail about the anatomy and physiology of the thyroid gland and endocrine system, and I talk about some of the conventional medical tests and treatments only on a basic level. The primary focus of this book is to show you how myself and other people with hyperthyroid conditions restored their health by taking a natural treatment approach, and how you can do the same.

A lot of the information in this book is based on my personal experience with Graves' disease, as well as what I've seen by working with other people with hyperthyroid and autoimmune hyperthyroid conditions since 2009. While a lot of this information is based on the experience of myself and my patients, just like any book, at times I will make references to other sources as well. Although I did spend time doing research for this book, please keep in mind that there hasn't been much research with regards to natural treatment methods and hyperthyroid conditions. This should be easy to understand when you realize that most research studies are actually conducted by the pharmaceutical companies.

So while there are numerous references of clinical studies in this book, a great deal of the information in this book is not based on hundreds of clinical studies on the effectiveness of natural treatment methods, but is instead based on my personal experience with Graves' disease, the experience of my patients, and the fact that we were born with our thyroid gland for a reason. As you know, we don't develop hyperthyroidism and Graves' disease due to a deficiency of radioactive iodine, methimazole, or propylthiouracil (PTU). This doesn't mean that some people don't need these conventional medical treatment methods, but to tell everyone with hyperthyroid conditions to either take antithyroid drugs and pray for a remission, or to obliterate their thyroid gland using radioactive iodine is in my opinion ludicrous.

Despite the lack of research out there, once you are done reading this book I don't think you'll find it difficult to understand how natural treatment methods might be able to restore your health. The reason for this is because a lot of what I discuss is based on common sense. This of course doesn't mean that everyone with hyperthyroidism can fully regain their health, but after reading this book you'll discover why most people with hyperthyroid conditions can greatly benefit from taking a natural treatment approach.

Here is a brief summary of the different chapters which are in this book:

Chapter 2: My Personal Story. In this chapter I discuss my personal experience with Graves' disease, and how I was skeptical about whether I would be able to restore my health through a natural treatment approach. I also briefly discuss how I began helping people with thyroid and autoimmune thyroid conditions.

Chapter 3: Hyperthyroidism vs. Graves' Disease: What's The Difference? In this chapter I discuss the difference between Graves' disease and other hyperthyroid conditions. The truth is that just about all of the information in this book can benefit people with any type of hyperthyroidism.

Chapter 4: Finding The Underlying Cause Of Your Condition. In this chapter I discuss how most endocrinologists and other types of medical doctors don't look for the actual cause of the hyperthyroid condition. On the other hand, the goal of a competent natural healthcare practitioner will be to find the underlying cause of your condition in an attempt to help you restore your health. This chapter will discuss some of the systems of the body which can lead to the development of hyperthyroidism.

Chapter 5: My True Feelings About Conventional Medical Treatment Methods. In this chapter I focus on conventional medical treatment methods. While many people might think I'm opposed to people taking antithyroid drugs and getting thyroid surgery, the truth is that I realize there is a time and place for these types of treatments.

Chapter 6: Do Natural Treatment Methods Provide A Permanent Cure? In this chapter I discuss whether natural treatment methods can provide a permanent cure for hyperthyroidism, or if they just provide a temporary solution.

Chapter 7: The Immune System Component Of Graves' Disease. In this chapter I discuss the importance of the immune system with regards to Graves' disease, and how conventional medical treatment does nothing to address the immune system component. I also discuss five factors which can lead to a compromised immune system.

Chapter 8: The Role That Stress Plays In The Development Of Hyperthyroidism. In this chapter I discuss how prolonged stress can potentially lead to the development of hyperthyroidism and Graves' disease, and how stress affects the adrenal glands. I also list 12 stress management tips to help better manage your stress.

Chapter 9: The Importance Of Proper Digestion In Restoring Your Health. In this chapter I discuss why it's important to have a properly functioning digestive system for anyone looking to restore their health, and I give seven tips to help improve your digestive health.

Chapter 10: The Immune-Gut Connection and Graves' Disease. In this chapter I discuss how having problems with the gut can be a factor in autoimmunity, thus leading to a condition such as Graves' disease.

Chapter 11: Hyperthyroid Diet Tips. In this chapter I give an actual example of a "hyperthyroid healing diet" you can follow, I give the pros and cons of an elimination diet, and I reveal five important rules anyone with hyperthyroidism should follow.

Chapter 12: Nutritional Supplements & Herbs For Hyperthyroidism & Graves' Disease. In this chapter I discuss some of the nutritional supplements and herbal remedies which can benefit people with hyperthyroidism.

Chapter 13: The Truth About Iodine And Hyperthyroidism. In this chapter I talk about the iodine controversy, and the risks and benefits associated with iodine supplementation for those with hyperthyroidism.

Chapter 14: Can Environmental Toxins Trigger Graves' Disease? In this chapter I discuss the impact of environmental toxins on our health, and how they can lead to an autoimmune thyroid condition such as Graves' disease. I talk about xenohormones, indoor and outdoor pollution, heavy metals, and I discuss what you can do about these environmental toxins.

Chapter 15: The Role of Infections In The Development of Graves' Disease. In this chapter I talk about the impact that infections can have on one's health. Numerous studies have linked certain infections with the development of hyperthyroidism and Graves' disease.

Chapter 16: How Big Of A Role Does Genetics Play? In this chapter I discuss how genetics alone doesn't determine whether someone will develop hyperthyroidism or Graves' disease, and how environmental factors usually play a greater role.

Chapter 17: Graves' Disease & Thyroid Antibodies. In this chapter I discuss the significance of the tests for thyroid antibodies and whether a natural treatment approach will help to lower these antibodies. I also talk about the radioactive iodine uptake test and whether or not it is necessary for people with hyperthyroidism to receive this test.

Chapter 18: 5 Reasons To Avoid Radioactive Iodine Treatment. In this chapter I discuss five reasons why radioactive iodine treatment should be avoided.

Chapter 19: The Risks Of Playing The Waiting Game. In this chapter I discuss the risk of relying solely on antithyroid drugs and hoping it will put you into a state of remission.

Chapter 20: Combining Natural Treatment Methods With Conventional Treatment Methods. In this chapter I discuss why it might be wise for some people to continue taking antithyroid medication while taking a natural treatment approach. I also discuss the herbs bugleweed and motherwort, and whether they can be safely used as substitutes for antithyroid drugs.

Chapter 21: Can Thyroid Nodules Be Treated Naturally? In this chapter I discuss some of the common causes of thyroid nodules, how natural treatment methods might be able to help with thyroid nodules, and I also list four situations when someone with thyroid nodules might want to consider using medical intervention. I also discuss when a thyroid biopsy is necessary, and what you need to know about radiofrequency ablation and thyroid nodules.

Chapter 22: Overcoming Thyroid Eye Disease. In this chapter I discuss how taking a natural treatment approach can potentially help someone who has thyroid eye disease, including the impact of diet and lifestyle on TED, and what supplements can be beneficial. I'll also discuss the benefits and risks associated with Tepezza.

Chapter 23: Natural Treatment Methods During Pregnancy & Lactation. In this chapter I discuss the different treatment options for women with hyperthyroidism who are pregnant or breastfeeding, along with the potential concerns of nutritional supplements and herbs.

Chapter 24: Can a Natural Treatment Approach Help With a Thyroid Storm? In this chapter I discuss the condition known as thyroid storm, whether or not natural treatment methods can help with this urgent situation, and how to prevent a thyroid storm from occurring in the first place.

Chapter 25: Overcoming Toxic Multinodular Goiter. In this chapter I talk about toxic multinodular goiter, including some of the common causes, and why people with this condition should consider taking a natural treatment approach.

Chapter 26: 5 Reasons Why You Shouldn't Self-Treat Your Hyperthyroid Condition. In this chapter I discuss why people with hyperthyroidism shouldn't self treat their condition, giving five specific reasons. Many people look to treat their condition naturally, and if this describes you, then you definitely will want to read this chapter carefully.

Chapter 27: Natural Treatment Methods Don't Cure Anything. In this chapter I talk about what the real goal of a natural treatment approach is, and how natural treatment methods don't cure hyperthyroidism, but instead strives to put the body into an optimal state of health.

Chapter 28: What Can You Do If Natural Treatment Methods Aren't Effective? In this chapter I discuss some of the reasons people might not receive good results when taking a natural treatment approach, and the different options people have when a natural treatment approach isn't effective, including low dose naltrexone and cholestyramine.

Chapter 29: The Keys To Maintaining Your Health. In this chapter I discuss how after restoring your health you can maintain a state of wellness for many years to come. I'll also let you know which supplements you can consider taking on a wellness basis.

Chapter 30: Consult With A Natural Healthcare Practitioner. In this chapter I discuss the importance of working with a natural healthcare practitioner who focuses on thyroid and autoimmune thyroid conditions. I also give some advice when it comes to choosing a natural healthcare practitioner.

Chapter 31: Formulate An Action Plan To Restore Your Health. In this chapter I discuss some things you can do right now to help restore your health, including four specific action steps.

Chapter 32: Additional Natural Thyroid Health Resources. This chapter provides some of the different resources, mostly free, to help you save your thyroid and regain your health. This includes the Save My Thyroid podcast, my Natural Endocrine Solutions website (www.naturalendocrinesolutions. com), my Natural Thyroid Doctor YouTube channel, and some other valuable resources.

Chapter 33: Twenty Three Questions You May Have About Natural Treatment Methods. In this Chapter I answer twenty three of the common questions people have about natural treatment methods. Here are just a few of the questions I answer:

- Should Gluten Be Avoided In People With Hyperthyroidism?
- Can Natural Treatment Methods Help People With Subclinical Hyperthyroidism?
- Can Goiter Be Decreased In People With Hyperthyroidism & Graves Disease?
- Can A Vegetarian Receive Good Results When Following A Natural Treatment Protocol?
- I Thought Most People With Hyperthyroidism Lose Weight. Why Am I Gaining Weight?
- What Can Be Done For Hair Loss Caused By Hyperthyroidism?

Reading This Book Can Change Your Life

I have had many people email me after visiting my website, listening to the Save My Thyroid podcast, or reading the first or second edition of this book, stating that the information I provided has changed their life.

I'm hoping the same thing will happen after you read the revised third edition of this book.

You should think of this book as an investment in your health, as not only can it help to restore your health with regards to your hyperthyroid condition, but it should also help with your overall health as well. With that being said, I would like to thank you for taking the time to read this book, and I'm confident that you will find the following information to be extremely valuable.

For access to the book references and resources, visit
savemythyroid.com/hyperbooknotes

CHAPTER 2

My Personal Story

Since graduating from chiropractic college in 1999 I had considered myself to be in a good state of health. Although I didn't eat a perfect diet upon graduating, I think it's safe to say that I ate better than most people, exercised regularly, obtained at least seven to eight hours of sleep each night, etc. But one day in 2008 I was walking into a retail store and saw one of those sit-down automated blood pressure machines. It had been a few months since I measured my blood pressure, and so I decided to get my blood pressure taken.

My blood pressure was fine, but I was shocked when the device revealed that my pulse rate was 90 beats per minute. Normally my pulse rate was in the mid 60's, and so I wasn't sure what was going on at the time. I immediately took my pulse rate manually, thinking that perhaps the machine wasn't working correctly. But sure enough, the manual readings were right around the same number.

The next few days I continued to monitor my pulse rate manually, and at any given time it was anywhere from 90 to 100 beats per minute, and at times higher than this. At the time I had also lost a lot of weight, but a few months before discovering the high pulse rate I followed a liver detoxification program and then continued eating well and restricting calories, and so I thought the weight loss might be due to my new regimen. It wasn't until after I discovered that I had a high pulse rate when I started linking this with the weight loss, and then I knew I had to get this checked out.

Off To The Medical Doctor I Went!

So I made a rare trip to a medical doctor, and after receiving the TSH and free T4 blood tests, I was told that I had a hyperthyroid condition. To be honest, I wasn't too concerned at the time, as I was relieved that I didn't have something more serious, such as cancer. On the other hand, being a natural healthcare practitioner I was familiar with hyperthyroidism, and I knew that radioactive iodine was commonly recommended by endocrinologists. Plus, as is the case with most people who have been diagnosed with any type of health condition, I of course did plenty of research online.

So when I visited an endocrinologist about one month later I was prepared for her to recommend radioactive iodine to obliterate my thyroid gland. When I went to the endocrinologist, she performed a thyroid examination, recommended additional blood tests (TSH, free T4 and T3, tests for thyroid antibodies, etc.), and she eventually diagnosed me with Graves' disease.

My goal here isn't to go into detail about the purpose of the different tests, as I mentioned in an earlier chapter that there are some good books out there which go into great detail about the radioactive iodine uptake test, thyroid blood tests, thyroid antibodies, etc. I will discuss some of these tests briefly in this book, but if you want to learn more about these tests then there are plenty of other resources available which discuss this information in greater detail. In Chapter 1 I also mentioned my free Foundations of Overcoming Hyperthyroidism Online Course. Once again, you can learn more about the online course by visiting savemythyroid.com/foundations.

You also might want to check out my podcast, Save My Thyroid, as well as the website www.naturalendocrinesolutions.com, which has hundreds of articles and blog posts related to thyroid health.

Fortunately the endocrinologist I saw was somewhat conservative and to my surprise she just told me that I should take methimazole and a beta blocker and hope my condition goes into remission. However, even before I saw this doctor I knew I was going to try taking a natural treatment approach. Being a natural healthcare practitioner, I knew that there had to be a cause behind my Graves' disease condition, and I also knew that taking antithyroid drugs or receiving radioactive iodine treatment might help to manage the hyperthyroid symptoms, but wouldn't do anything to address the cause.

Even I Was Skeptical About Natural Treatment Methods

Even though I'm a natural healthcare practitioner and made up my mind that I would take a natural treatment approach in an attempt to reverse my Graves' disease condition, this doesn't mean I wasn't skeptical. Without question I had my doubts about whether a natural treatment approach would restore my health. Quite frankly, at the time I would have been happy with continuous natural symptom management. I just wanted to avoid having to take prescription drugs, and definitely wanted to avoid receiving radioactive iodine.

At first I was planning to self-treat my condition. After all, while I didn't have much experience dealing with people who had hyperthyroidism at the time, in the past I did see a lot of people with hypothyroidism, fibromyalgia and other chronic conditions in my practice, and so I did wonder why I couldn't simply self-treat my condition? But after thinking it through, I decided to play it safe and I consulted with another natural healthcare professional who focused on thyroid conditions. And even though she didn't have much experience dealing with Graves' disease at that time, speaking with her turned out to be one of the best decisions I ever made.

The most worrisome symptoms I had were the high pulse rate and heart palpitations I experienced, although I also had lost a lot of weight (I went from 182 pounds to 140 pounds), and I had a voracious appetite. I also experienced tremors, especially when getting blood tests, as when they were drawing the blood I found it difficult to keep my arm from shaking. After only a few weeks of following a natural treatment protocol I began noticing a decrease in my heart rate and palpitations. A few months later my palpitations were just about gone, my pulse rate normalized, the tremors were gone, and I had gained a lot of the weight I lost back (fortunately not all of it!). The only symptom which remained was the voracious appetite, although this eventually disappeared as well.

As for the blood tests, a few months after beginning the natural treatment approach my thyroid blood tests began to improve. There is no better feeling than the one I had when I received my first follow up blood tests and saw some positive changes. Gradually my thyroid hormones and thyroid stimulating immunoglobulins decreased. It took awhile before the thyroid stimulating hormone (TSH) started to increase, which is typical with hyperthyroidism.

Overall it took approximately nine months before my thyroid blood tests became completely normal without having to rely on any antithyroid herbs, although at the time I still wasn't sure if they would remain normal. I also received additional "alternative" tests which I will discuss in this book (i.e. saliva test), and these tests also greatly improved. I should also add that everyone is different, as while some people with hyperthyroidism will notice positive changes in their thyroid markers one or two months after starting a natural treatment approach, for some people it will take longer.

The Student Becomes The Teacher

After seeing how effective natural treatment methods were in helping with my autoimmune thyroid condition, I developed a passion to help other people with hyperthyroidism and Graves' disease, as well as other thyroid and autoimmune thyroid conditions (i.e. Hashimoto's thyroiditis). After all, I knew there were thousands of people each year who had their thyroid gland obliterated through radioactive iodine treatment or removed through surgery, and I felt that many of these people could be helped through natural treatment methods. The problem is that most people with hyperthyroidism aren't even aware that a natural treatment approach might be able to help them.

So in 2009 I began helping people who had Graves' disease, toxic multi-nodular goiter, Hashimoto's thyroiditis, and other thyroid/autoimmune thyroid conditions who were interested in using a natural treatment approach to restore their health. However, even though I've worked with a lot of people with Hashimoto's over the years, as of writing the third edition of my book, approximately 85% of my patients have hyperthyroidism. And the main reason for this is because I'm one of the few natural healthcare practitioners who has a great deal of experience working with those who have hyperthyroidism.

In addition to being a licensed doctor of chiropractic, after my own hyperthyroid journey I began receiving additional training, as I'm a Certified Nutrition Specialist℠, a certified clinical nutritionist, I received my Masters in Nutrition degree in 2014, and I became certified through the Institute for Functional Medicine in 2016. I also have received a certificate in practical herbal therapy from the Australian College of Phytotherapy. Since I began this venture I've been surprised as to how many people have expressed interest in using natural treatment methods to restore their health.

In 2010 I created the website naturalendocrinesolutions.com. This website not only focuses on natural treatment solutions for hyperthyroidism and Graves' disease, but hypothyroidism and Hashimoto's thyroiditis as well. In addition, I created a guide entitled "The 6 Steps On How To Treat Graves' Disease and Hashimoto's Thyroiditis Naturally", and offer this guide for free on my website. The guide contains some great content, and in addition to this guide I have created a lot of quality content on the website, as there are hundreds of articles and blog posts related to thyroid and autoimmune thyroid conditions, many of which focus on hyperthyroidism.

Although I had thousands of people visiting my website each month shortly after creating it, I still felt like there were many people with hyperthyroidism who weren't aware of the benefits of natural treatment methods. And so I decided to write this book, figuring a lot of people might not come across my website, but they just might discover my book and learn how taking a natural treatment approach can possibly benefit them.

The first edition of this book was published in 2011, and then I came out with a revised edition in 2013. Over the last decade I have learned a great deal of additional information not only through the education I've received and the research I've conducted, but also through my personal experience. During this time I have helped thousands of people with hyperthyroidism and Graves' disease avoid radioactive iodine and thyroid surgery through my website, book, podcast, and program for hyperthyroid patients, and I figured it was a good time to update this book for a third time.

In 2021 I launched the "Save My Thyroid" podcast (savemythyroid. com), which helps people with hyperthyroidism and Hashimoto's save their thyroid. While many of the episodes can benefit both people with hyperthyroidism and Hashimoto's, if you browse through the episodes you'll notice that there definitely is an emphasis on hyperthyroidism. And the reason for this is because there is no shortage of podcasts that focus on hypothyroidism, but as of writing the third edition of this book there isn't one that focuses on hyperthyroidism. With that being said, let's move onto the next chapter and begin to discover how a natural treatment approach can help you regain your health.

For access to the book references and resources, visit
savemythyroid.com/hyperbooknotes

CHAPTER 3

Hyperthyroidism vs. Graves' Disease: What's The Difference?

THROUGHOUT THIS BOOK you'll notice that at times I mention both "hyperthyroidism and Graves' disease", rather than pertain to them both at the same time by simply saying "hyperthyroid conditions" or "hyperthyroidism". Graves' disease is the most common hyperthyroid condition, and about 90% of people with hyperthyroidism have Graves' disease. On the other hand, there are people with hyperthyroid conditions who don't have Graves' disease.

What I'm basically doing in this book is separately referring to 1) hyperthyroid conditions without an autoimmune component, and 2) Graves' disease, which is an autoimmune hyperthyroid condition. Of course one can't always completely rely on the tests which are routinely performed on people with hyperthyroidism. As a result, even if you have been diagnosed as having hyperthyroidism but not Graves' disease, this doesn't mean you have a healthy immune system.

So even if you have been diagnosed with hyperthyroidism and the tests for thyroid antibodies (TSI, TPO etc.) were negative, as well as the radioactive iodine uptake test, most of the information in this book still applies to you as well, even the chapters which focus on "Graves' disease". So yes, there are differences between non-autoimmune hyperthyroidism and Graves' disease, and other hyperthyroid conditions as well (i.e. toxic multinodular goiter, subclinical hyperthyroidism). But regardless of what type of hyperthyroid condition you have, I do strongly recommend for you to read this entire book word for word, and not to skip over the chapters which focus primarily on Graves' disease.

The same concept applies to my original website (naturalendocrinesolutions. com), as if you visit it you will notice there are separate pages for "hyperthyroid conditions" and "Graves Disease". You'll also notice some articles I have written and videos I created focus on hyperthyroid conditions, while others focus on Graves' disease. In most cases I do this for "niching and keyword purposes", as someone who has been diagnosed with Graves' disease will find a headline with the word "Graves' disease" more appealing than hyperthyroidism, while reverse is true with someone who has been diagnosed with hyperthyroidism which doesn't have an autoimmune component. Similarly, when searching online, some people use the search terms "hyperthyroidism", while others use "Graves' disease".

And just as is the case with my website, with my podcast, Save My Thyroid, there are different episodes which focus on "hyperthyroidism", and others which focus on "Graves' disease". But once again, a lot of the content will benefit people with any type of hyperthyroid condition.

In any case, whether you have Graves' disease or non-autoimmune hyperthyroidism, I expect you to find most of the information in this book to be valuable. And so if you have a hyperthyroid condition but haven't been diagnosed with Graves' disease, keep in mind that false negative antibodies are possible, and even if this isn't the case, there is always the possibility of developing Graves' disease (or a different autoimmune condition) in the future. Because of this it's a good idea to read all of the information in this book which focuses on Graves' disease and follow the advice given so you not only will restore your thyroid health, but you will also optimize the health of your immune system, gut microbiome, adrenal glands, and other bodily systems so that you hopefully will never develop an autoimmune thyroid condition.

What Exactly Is Graves' Disease?

I assume that most people reading this already know what Graves' disease is, but at the same time most probably don't have a true understanding of this condition. Once again, the goal of this book isn't to get deep into the physiology behind hyperthyroid conditions, but I do think it's important to understand some of the basics, and why some people develop conditions such as Graves' disease.

One of the concepts I'll constantly bring up in the upcoming chapters is that Graves' disease isn't a thyroid condition, but instead is an autoimmune condition which affects the thyroid gland. There are many different types of autoimmune conditions, and the main characteristic they share is that they involve autoantibodies. In other words, each type of autoimmune condition involves a specific type of antibody, which in turn attacks a specific part of the body.

For example, Graves' disease involves antibodies which attack the TSH receptors. In order for the thyroid gland to secrete thyroid hormone, TSH, which is a pituitary hormone, needs to bind to these receptors. When TSH binds to these receptors, thyroid hormone is secreted. So think of the TSH receptor antibodies as taking the place of TSH, and so essentially they stimulate the TSH receptors, which in turn causes the excess production of thyroid hormone.

So how does this differ from an autoimmune condition such as Hashimoto's thyroiditis? Well, Hashimoto's thyroiditis involves different types of thyroid antibodies. Whereas Graves' disease is associated with TSH receptor antibodies, Hashimoto's thyroiditis is characterized by having thyroperoxidase (TPO) antibodies and/or thyroglobulin antibodies. Both of these antibodies directly attack different parts of the thyroid gland, and it's the destruction of this gland which reduces the output of thyroid hormone, resulting in a hypothyroid condition. Keep in mind that many people with Graves' disease will also have TPO and/or thyroglobulin antibodies.

How Does Graves' Disease Develop?

I'll talk about some of the different ways in which Graves' disease develops in different chapters of this book. Most people who develop Graves' disease do have a genetic predisposition for this condition. But as you'll learn later on, just having a genetic marker doesn't mean you will develop Graves' disease. Many people who have a genetic marker for Graves' disease never develop this condition. And the same concept holds true for other autoimmune conditions as well. In most cases, lifestyle and environmental factors trigger the genetics, which causes a condition such as Graves' disease.

In the next chapter I'm going to go into greater detail about the underlying causes of hyperthyroidism. And then later on I'll also talk more about the immune system component of Graves' disease. By the time you're finished reading this book I hope you'll have a better understanding of your condition, and realize that in most cases, conventional medical treatment methods such as radioactive iodine treatment and thyroid surgery aren't necessary to receive.

Chapter Summary

- Although most people with hyperthyroidism have Graves' Disease, there are different types of hyperthyroid conditions.
- Just because you haven't been diagnosed with Graves' Disease doesn't mean you have a healthy immune system. And some people who are diagnosed with non-autoimmune hyperthyroidism will eventually develop Graves disease.
- Whether you have non-autoimmune hyperthyroidism or Graves' Disease, I expect you to find most of the information in this book to be useful.
- Remember that Graves' Disease is not a thyroid condition, but instead is an autoimmune condition which affects the thyroid gland.
- Graves' Disease involves TSH receptor antibodies, which attack the TSH receptors, thus resulting in the excess production of thyroid hormone

For access to the book references and resources, visit
savemythyroid.com/hyperbooknotes

CHAPTER 4

Finding The Underlying Cause Of Your Condition

WHEN I FIRST BEGAN helping others with thyroid and autoimmune thyroid conditions in 2009, one of the first people I consulted with was a 29-year old female patient (we'll call her Rita) who developed hypothyroidism as a result of receiving radioactive iodine treatment. She was 22 years old when she made a routine visit to her medical doctor, and her blood tests revealed that she had subclinical hyperthyroidism, as she had low TSH levels. Even though she wasn't experiencing any symptoms at the time, and her thyroid hormone levels were normal, she was referred to an endocrinologist, where it was recommended that she receive radioactive iodine treatment.

Like most people who are diagnosed with hyperthyroidism, Rita didn't know much about her condition. She also didn't realize the consequences of receiving radioactive iodine, and was convinced by the endocrinologist that this would be the best option to "cure" her condition. So even though she wasn't experiencing any symptoms at the time, she went ahead and received the radioactive iodine, and as a result had to take thyroid hormone replacement on a daily basis.

One thing which has puzzled me is how most endocrinologists and other types of medical doctors don't look for the underlying cause of hyper-thyroidism and Graves' disease. Whenever someone is diagnosed with hyperthyroidism, they are either told to 1) receive radioactive iodine to obliterate the thyroid gland, 2) get thyroid surgery, or 3) take antithyroid drugs and essentially pray that the condition goes into remission. Very rarely do they try to find the underlying cause and then attempt to address this cause.

For example, it's no secret that everyone who has Graves' disease has a compromised immune system. I know this, you know this, and your endocrinologist or general medical practitioner knows this as well. Yet, nothing is ever done to address the immune system component. Telling someone to receive radioactive iodine or to take antithyroid medication might help with the symptoms, but these treatment methods will do absolutely nothing for the immune system. There are numerous factors that can trigger the autoimmune response associated with Graves' disease, including stressed out adrenal glands, environmental toxins, and infections.

But these other factors are never looked at, as the focus is on the thy-roid gland itself, which is rarely the direct cause of the condition. Sure, evaluating and treating the thyroid gland is important, but if one only focuses on the thyroid gland itself, then it shouldn't be a surprise why most endocrinologists label Graves' disease as being incurable. Because the truth is that while conventional medical treatment is sometimes necessary for this autoimmune thyroid condition, if the underlying cause isn't detected and then addressed, then one obviously won't be able to restore their health.

Why Do Some People Develop Hyperthyroidism?

Now you know that it's usually not the malfunctioning thyroid gland itself which is the root cause of the problem. One needs to look at the adrenals, gut microbiome, and other triggers/underlying imbalances. But what exactly causes adrenal problems, gut issues, toxic overload, etc.? I focus on some of the primary factors which can lead to these later on in this book, but for now let's briefly take a look at some of the factors which can lead to the development of hyperthyroidism:

Factor #1: Poor diet. Eating healthy is important when dealing with any chronic health condition. And while eating a healthy diet alone won't always reverse one's hyperthyroid condition, if someone eats inflammatory foods on a regular basis it will be very difficult to heal.

So at this point you might be wondering what foods you should eat? I'll talk about diet more in Chapter 11, but I will say here that there isn't a single diet that fits everyone perfectly. And if after reading Chapter 11 you decide that you want even more information related to diet and hyperthyroidism you'll definitely want to check out my book the "Hyperthyroid Healing Diet", which will be released in the first quarter of 2024. You can learn more by visiting hyperthyroidhealingdietbook.com.

Factor #2: An inability to handle stress. While most people know that stress can cause a lot of health problems, most don't truly understand the impact that chronic stress can have on one's health over a period of many months or years. The human body was designed to handle acute stress situations, but it can't effectively deal with prolonged, chronic stress. But it's not the chronic stress itself which causes the problem, but rather the inability to handle this type of stress.

So a person who deals with chronic stress and does a poor job of managing it will be more susceptible to developing these conditions when compared to someone who has better stress handling skills. The person with poor stress handling skills has a good chance of developing problems with their adrenal glands, which can affect immunity, digestion, as well as the thyroid gland itself. As a result, over a period of time a person with compromised adrenals can eventually develop an autoimmune thyroid condition, such as Graves' disease. I'm not suggesting that this alone causes Graves' disease, but I don't think it's a coincidence that most people with hyperthyroidism and Graves' disease have problems with their adrenals.

Factor #3: Disrupted gut microbiome. I realize it's difficult for many people to make the connection between gut dysbiosis and thyroid health. By the way, gut dysbiosis is the medical term for an imbalance in the gut flora. In any case, there are numerous ways in which gut dysbiosis can lead to hyperthyroidism and Graves' disease.

First of all, more and more healthcare professionals are becoming aware of the connection between an increase in intestinal permeability (leaky gut) and autoimmune conditions such as Graves' disease. This doesn't just include chiropractors and naturopathic doctors, but many medical doctors are also aware that leaky gut syndrome is a true condition, and seems to be a factor in the development of autoimmune conditions.[5] I'll be dedicating a separate chapter to this, and after you read this information you'll have a better understanding as to how problems with the gut can cause an autoimmune condition such as Graves' disease to develop.

But even if someone doesn't have a leaky gut, other gut issues can potentially cause or contribute to conditions such as hyperthyroidism. For example, if someone has an absorption problem, then this can lead to nutritional deficiencies. And certain deficiencies of vitamins and minerals can potentially cause hyperthyroidism to develop, or can affect the immune system and/or other bodily systems and make someone more susceptible to developing an autoimmune thyroid condition such as Graves' disease.

H. Pylori is a bacteria in the stomach which can interfere with the production of hydrochloric acid, thus leading to nutritional deficiencies. A few studies have linked H. Pylori to autoimmune thyroid conditions.[6,7] These studies suggest that there is a strong correlation between H. Pylori and Graves' disease. H. Pylori is a gut bacteria that is easy to acquire, but difficult to eradicate.

Now to be fair, there is controversy over whether H. pylori should be eradicated in the absence of certain gastrointestinal symptoms (i.e. heartburn, reflux), but I can say that over the years I've had patients get into remission after following a natural antimicrobial protocol for H. pylori. This doesn't mean that whenever someone with Graves' disease tests positive for H. pylori that it's the trigger, but it very well can be.

Factor #4: Environmental toxins. I just mentioned earlier how it's impossible to completely eliminate the stress from your life. Similarly, it is also unlikely that you will be able to avoid exposure to all of the environmental toxins. There are thousands of environmental toxins we're exposed to, and many of them are in the foods we eat and the products we buy.

There's a book called "The Autoimmune Epidemic", which talks about how different environmental toxins can affect the immune system and possibly lead to the development of autoimmune conditions.[8] It makes sense when you think about it, as over the last few decades we have been exposed to more and more environmental toxins, and the rate of autoimmune thyroid conditions such as Graves' disease have also increased. Obviously other factors are involved, but one can't overlook the impact of all the toxic chemicals we're constantly being exposed to on a daily basis.

I'm going to talk more about detoxification in a different chapter, but a good book I recommend for everyone to read is called "Clean, Green, and Lean", which was written by the late Dr. Walter Crinnion. Dr. Crinnion was an expert in environmental medicine, as he was a naturopathic doctor who practiced for over 30 years. Dr. Crinnion was my instructor in the "Detoxification and Biotransformation Pathways and Imbalances" course I took during my Masters in Nutrition program.

Even before being mentored by him I felt like I had a great deal of knowledge in detoxification, as I've been putting my patients on detoxification programs for many years. But after going through his class I gained an even greater amount of knowledge on this topic. Just to let you know, Dr. Crinnion's book is targeted towards people looking to lose weight, and of course many people with hyperthyroidism have the opposite problem. However, the main purpose of his book is to show you how to reduce your exposure to environmental toxins, which of course everyone can benefit from.

After all, when you consider all of the different environmental toxins we're exposed to on a daily basis, including xenohormones, heavy metals, pesticides, volatile organic compounds, glyphosate, and many other toxins, it's not a surprise that many people have all of these chronic health conditions. There are thousands of toxins we're exposed to, and just as our adrenals weren't designed to handle the chronic stress most people deal with on a daily basis, our liver and immune system weren't designed to handle all of these toxins. And most people who try to detoxify their body on their own aren't doing a good enough job. Heck, after going through Dr. Crinnion's class I realized that I could do a better job of helping my patients to reduce their toxic load, and the same thing can be said for most healthcare practitioners.

Factor #5: Infections. Certain bacteria, viruses, and other infections can compromise the immune system, and can potentially trigger an autoimmune response. I'll be talking about this in greater detail in Chapter 15, but some of the different pathogens which have been associated with Graves' disease include Borrelia burgdorferi (the bacteria involved in Lyme disease), Hepatitis C, Yersinia enterocolitica, H. Pylori, and Epstein-Barr. Keep in mind that many people are exposed to these and other pathogens. Despite this, the majority of these people don't develop an autoimmune condition such as Graves' disease.

So why do some people who are exposed to infections develop an auto-immune condition? A genetic predisposition to autoimmunity does play a role. As a result, someone with a genetic marker for Graves' disease who gets exposed to one of these potentially pathogenic microbes is more likely to develop this condition than someone without a genetic predisposition. However, and as you'll learn shortly, just having a genetic marker for Graves' disease doesn't mean that someone will develop this condition, even if they're exposed to one or more of these infections.

The health of the immune system plays a big role in whether these infections will trigger an autoimmune response. And this is the case with many different bacteria, viruses, parasites, etc. For example, two people might be exposed to the same virus, and while one person might become sick for days or weeks, the other person won't develop any symptoms. And a big reason for this has to do with the health of the person's immune system.

Similarly, someone can have a genetic predisposition to Graves' disease, and upon exposure to one of these microbes they might not develop this condition if they have a healthy immune system. Another scenario is that the infection may not trigger an autoimmune response right away, but might lie dormant for a period of months or years, and can eventually lead to the development of an autoimmune condition such as Graves' disease. Once again, I'll talk more about infections in Chapter 15.

Factor #6: Genetics. Although genetics can play a role in the development of non-autoimmune hyperthyroidism, or an autoimmune condition such as Graves' disease, the good news is that it does not play as big of a role as many people think. More and more studies show that people with genetic tendencies towards certain conditions may have such conditions triggered by external factors,[9] such as the five I just discussed. So rather than worry about whether your condition is caused by factors you can't control, you might as well focus on those factors which you do have control over.

So these are some of the common factors which can lead to the development of hyperthyroidism and Graves' disease. Since most endocrinologists label these conditions as being incurable, it shouldn't surprise you that they don't focus on these factors. However, for any competent natural healthcare professional, looking into these lifestyle and environmental factors is important when trying to restore the health of someone with a hyperthyroid condition.

While there can be other factors which can cause or contribute to the development of a thyroid or autoimmune thyroid condition, in many cases, focusing on the first four factors I discussed in this chapter will help to restore the person's health. In other words, if someone eats a healthy, anti-inflammatory diet, has healthy adrenal glands, a healthy gut microbiome, and a lower toxic burden, then this in turn will usually lead to a healthy immune system, and in many cases will help to restore the health of the person with hyperthyroidism. That being said, sometimes other factors need to be addressed, such as infections, estrogen dominance, toxic mold, etc.

The Challenge of Reversing Hyperthyroidism

It shouldn't be a surprise that restoring the health of someone who has hyperthyroidism is not a quick and easy process, and therefore will take some time. Some people will try to self-treat their condition, but it really is a good idea to consult with a competent natural healthcare practitioner, as such a person will look for the underlying cause of the problem. Once they determine the cause they will then put together an individualized natural treatment protocol to help restore the person's health.

This will no doubt include modifying some of the lifestyle and environmental factors I briefly discussed before. So if you do a poor job of managing the stress in your life, a competent natural healthcare practitioner will help you to develop better stress handling skills while helping you to restore the health of the adrenal glands. If you have a leaky gut then they will help to restore the health of your gut microbiome, which includes balancing the gut flora and repairing the intestinal permeability problem.

If nutritional deficiencies are the problem, then in addition to healing the gut they should also encourage you to eat better, recommend the appropriate nutritional supplements for you to take, etc. With regards to environmental toxins, a natural healthcare practitioner will give recommendations to reduce your exposure to these toxins, while at the same time help you do things to assist with the elimination of these toxins from your body.

Being a natural healthcare professional I'm of course biased, and therefore recommend for most people who have hyperthyroidism to consult with a natural healthcare practitioner who has experience working with hyperthyroid patients. After all, antithyroid drugs can be important to take on a temporary basis, but they don't do anything to address any of the factors I've discussed, and radioactive iodine treatment and thyroid surgery should usually be a last resort. When you think about it, there really isn't much to lose by speaking with an expert, but there is a lot to potentially gain. Either way, in order for anyone with hyperthyroidism to restore their health they must take responsibility for their health.

Chapter Summary

- Most endocrinologists and other types of medical doctors don't look for the underlying cause of hyperthyroidism.
- Conventional medical treatment methods typically do nothing for the underlying cause of the problem
- The malfunctioning thyroid gland itself usually isn't the root cause of the problem
- Other underling imbalances such as compromised adrenals, gut dybiosis, and an increased toxic load usually cause or contribute to the development of the condition.
- Six factors which can cause hyperthyroidism include 1) poor diet, 2) an inability to handle stress, 3) a disrupted gut microbiome, 4) environmental toxins, 5) infections, and 6) genetics.
- Restoring the health of someone who has hyperthyroidism is not a quick and easy process

For access to the book references and resources, visit
savemythyroid.com/hyperbooknotes

CHAPTER 5

My True Feelings About Conventional Medical Treatment Methods

SOME PEOPLE WILL no doubt perceive this book as a widespread criticism of conventional medicine. After all, this book focuses a great deal on how many people receive radioactive iodine unnecessarily, and how antithyroid drugs don't do anything for the cause of the hyperthyroid condition. Even though I do think that many people who choose conventional medical treatment methods can benefit from taking a natural treatment approach, I also realize that conventional medicine does have its place.

While some natural healthcare practitioners are strongly opposed to conventional medicine, I wish that both natural healthcare professionals and medical doctors could work together, rather than fight one another. Without question there are a lot of things I don't agree with when it comes to conventional medical treatment, and the same thing can be said when it comes to how most medical doctors think of natural treatment methods. I don't think there's anything wrong with different types of doctors disagreeing with one another, but I do wish that more medical doctors would have an open mind towards alternative treatment methods.

My Feelings About The Pharmaceutical Companies

There is no question that prescription drugs save many lives, and that antithyroid drugs are important for many people with hyperthyroidism and Graves' disease. On the other hand, many people take prescription drugs unnecessarily. So does this mean I'm opposed to the pharmaceutical companies? Although I definitely don't agree that drugs are the solution in most cases, they too have their place and are important at times. Plus, we also need to look at the business side of things.

The truth is that the pharmaceutical companies do a wonderful job of marketing their products both to medical doctors and to the consumer. In fact, many patients visit their medical doctor and ask for specific prescription drugs they see on television or read about on the Internet. This is perhaps the main reason why most people choose medication over natural alternatives, as we are being constantly inundated by commercials and online advertising about these medications, while many people aren't even aware of the benefits of natural treatment methods. While the pharmaceutical companies do a great job of marketing their product, most natural healthcare practitioners don't spend much time marketing their practices, as they're too busy taking care of their patients.

Of course the same concept holds true with most medical doctors with regards to marketing their practices, as most medical doctors, as well as other types of healthcare practitioners, don't know much about marketing their business, as their primary goal is to help patients. This of course is how it should be, although the fact is that to succeed in any business, marketing plays a very important role. The point I'm trying to make is that the success of the drug industry doesn't have much to do with the safety and effectiveness of prescription drugs, but instead can be credited to their astute marketing. Again, this isn't meant to criticize the industry, but is just meant to demonstrate what type of impact strong marketing can have.

A recent example related to thyroid health is Tepezza, which is a medication for thyroid eye disease that has been available in the United States since 2020. I was surprised when I recently saw a commercial for Tepezza, but I probably shouldn't have been surprised, as it's quite expensive, and therefore very profitable. Now to be fair, I've had a few Graves' disease patients take Tepezza and it helped with their eye bulging. But just like any conventional treatment, there are potential side effects, and it doesn't do anything to address the underlying cause of the condition. I'll talk more about Tepezza in Chapter 22.

The Role Of Credibility Factors In Choosing Conventional Medical Treatment

Of course credibility also plays a big role in people's decision to choose medical treatment over alternative care. As a whole, medical doctors are more credible than natural healthcare professionals. Many people assume that because medical doctors go to medical school for many years and then spend many more years doing their residency that they have a greater amount of knowledge when compared to natural healthcare practitioners.

I'm not arguing that most medical doctors are very knowledgeable in the field of medicine, but many natural healthcare professionals receive an equivalent amount of training. For example, to become a chiropractor I received my bachelor's degree, spent an additional two years completing the prerequisite classes for chiropractic school, and then spent an additional four years in chiropractic college. The big difference is that most chiropractors complete their internship at the same time as taking their classes. In other words, during the last two years of school I took 24 credit hours per quarter and at the same time I was also required to see patients as part of my internship.

On the other hand, medical doctors go through medical school and then complete their residency. So while both medical doctors and chiropractors obviously receive a different type of training, the duration is very similar. And the same concept holds true for some other natural healthcare professionals, such as naturopathic physicians.

My goal isn't to take away any of the credibility of medical doctors, but it's to simply prove that many natural healthcare practitioners receive a sufficient amount of training as well. As I mentioned before, it would be great if more medical doctors and natural healthcare practitioners worked together, as this would benefit everyone. One thing it would accomplish is to give natural healthcare professionals more credibility, although many people are already choosing alternative care over conventional medical treatment.

But while I'm of course biased towards alternative treatment options, there are times when I do refer people to a medical doctor, and I do know that some medical doctors will refer their patients to natural healthcare practitioners. The problem is that it's rare for this to happen, and so many people who can benefit from seeing an alternative healthcare practitioner miss out because they aren't advised about natural treatment methods by their medical doctors. And the opposite holds true as well, as some people become turned off towards natural healthcare practitioners because some of these doctors claim that they can cure every condition, and will never refer a patient to a medical doctor under any set of circumstances.

Do I see this pattern changing anytime soon? Probably not, as while more medical doctors are becoming open minded towards functional medicine,

I still think it will be a long time before both medical doctors and natural healthcare practitioners work together on a regular basis.

Most People Are Looking For a "Quick Fix"

Even though our bodies have an amazing ability to heal, this takes time to happen, but most people are looking for a "quick fix" to their problem. There are some people who realize that prescription drugs are in many cases just covering up the symptoms, but they are fine with this. They don't have any interest in restoring their health.

If their thyroid gland is malfunctioning, then they are perfectly fine with taking thyroid medication, even if it's on a prolonged basis. If their cholesterol is high, then they see nothing wrong with taking statins (cholesterol-lowering medication) to provide a quick solution, rather than trying to get to the root cause of the problem. In other words, many people don't want to restore their health, even when this is possible.

On the other hand, many people don't want to take drugs to manage their symptoms when they know there is the possibility of having their health restored naturally. Other people don't mind taking medication such as antithyroid drugs on a temporary basis, but they still want to look for the underlying cause of the condition. This book is mainly aimed at these people.

While I of course would love for everyone with a hyperthyroid condition to read this book, the truth is that the only people who will read this book will be those who are open-minded towards a natural treatment approach. While more and more people are choosing natural treatment methods, there still are many who continue to choose conventional medical treatment methods due to many of the factors I discussed in this chapter.

Getting Medical Doctors To Open Their Minds Towards "Alternative Treatment Options" Is No Easy Task

While more and more consumers are choosing alternative healthcare, the same can be said about some medical doctors. Although most medical doctors still focus their practices on conventional medical treatments, some are becoming more aware of the benefits of functional medicine. Part of this most likely has to do with them realizing that more and more of their patients are looking for alternative options. So even though medical doctors don't receive training in medical school about nutritional supplements and herbs, many people don't realize this, and so they will approach their medical doctor and ask them about the safety and effectiveness of certain supplements and herbs. As a result, some medical doctors are becoming more open minded and are attempting to learn more about some of the more common nutritional supplements and herbs being sold on the market.

As for whether it's realistic to change the opinion of medical doctors and to get them to realize the benefits of alternative healthcare, in most cases this will be extremely difficult to accomplish. It would of course give me great pleasure to have endocrinologists read this book and realize that there are other options besides antithyroid drugs and radioactive iodine. And while some endocrinologists and other types of medical doctors who read this will be open minded to the information presented in this book, I expect most medical doctors not to be receptive to this material. But then again, even if this book causes a few endocrinologists to change their approach when it comes to recommending antithyroid medication or RAI then this would be wonderful.

In summary, both conventional medicine and alternative healthcare offer certain benefits. And while it would be great if most conventional medical doctors and natural healthcare practitioners would work together, I don't see this happening anytime soon. Although more medical doctors are becoming receptive to alternative treatment methods, many medical doctors still remain opposed to natural healthcare.

Chapter Summary

- Although I think many people who choose conventional treatment methods would benefit from a natural treatment approach, I also realize that conventional medicine has its place.
- Even though many people do need to take antithyroid drugs on a temporary basis, as well as other medication, many people take prescription drugs unnecessarily.
- Credibility plays a big role in people choosing medical doctors over natural healthcare practitioners, as most people perceive medical doctors as being more credible.
- Even though our bodies have an amazing ability to heal, it takes time for this to happen, but most people are looking for a "quick fix".
- While more and more people are turning towards alternative treatment methods, some medical doctors are also becoming more open minded towards functional medicine.

For access to the book references and resources, visit
savemythyroid.com/hyperbooknotes

CHAPTER 6

Do Natural Treatment Methods Provide A Permanent Cure?

WHEN CHARLIE WAS DIAGNOSED with Graves' disease, he was told by his endocrinologist to take methimazole to help manage the symptoms. His endocrinologist's plan was to have him take the medication for about 18 months, and hope that it would put him into a state of remission. Although some people respond well while taking the antithyroid drugs, Charlie just didn't feel good when taking the methimazole. As a result, his endocrinologist recommended that he take PTU instead, which he did, but he still didn't feel right. Both medications did control the hyperthyroid symptoms, but he just didn't "feel like himself" while taking either one of them.

So Charlie decided to give a natural treatment approach a try, and began noticing a big difference in his symptoms after only five weeks of following the protocol. And while after three months he still had a depressed TSH and elevated thyroid hormones, the thyroid hormones had decreased a great deal, and he told me he felt the best that he had in years. Before beginning the natural treatment approach Charlie ate a lot of refined foods and sugars, and didn't do a good job of managing his stress. While working with me he ate much better, took certain supplements for additional nutritional support, and developed better stress handling skills.

However, once he started feeling great he began eating refined foods and sugars again (he did continue to do a good job of managing his stress). While this is fine when done in moderation after restoring one's health, Charlie began eating these foods more and more frequently, and then one day he contacted me because he noticed his resting pulse rate was high again (although not as high as it was when he initially saw me), and he also began experiencing heart palpitations. He was upset because once the symptoms subsided he thought he would be able to stray from the diet without any consequences, but while most people can indulge every now and then after restoring their health, while you are trying to heal you want to be more strict with the diet and lifestyle.

More Than Just "Natural" Symptom Management

When I talk about using natural treatment methods for hyperthyroidism, you may wonder if taking a natural treatment approach can actually cure your condition, or will it just put your condition into a temporary state of remission? Before I answer this question, I first want to say that some people think of natural treatment methods as a "natural way" of managing the symptoms, and don't think of these treatment methods as doing anything for the actual cause of the condition. I can tell you from my personal experience that a genuine natural treatment approach should do more than just naturally manage the symptoms, as the goal isn't to take herbs such as bugleweed and motherwort on a permanent basis. And the same concept applies to other supplements and herbs that are needed, as the goal is to restore the person's health so they don't need to rely on medication, as well as most nutritional supplements and herbs.

But as for whether natural treatment methods can truly cure hyperthyroidism, including an autoimmune thyroid condition such as Graves' disease, it's necessary to understand what the difference is between a cure and a state of remission. Most of us are familiar with a condition such as cancer being in a state of remission, and we understand cancer in remission as not actually being permanently cured, but instead the condition is under control and is essentially in a "dormant" state. In other words, someone who is in remission from a certain type of cancer still supposedly has the cancer, but it's not in its "active" form.

In fact, I have a friend who was diagnosed with a type of leukemia a number of years ago. He took a fairly new type of medication at the time, and it not only controlled his symptoms, but over the last few years his leukemia has no longer been detectable on his blood tests. Despite this the doctors won't label him as being cured, but instead he has been told that he is in a state of remission. To put it another way, if he were to walk into another doctor's office who didn't know he was diagnosed with leukemia, they most likely wouldn't be able to tell he had such a condition, as all of the tests would come out negative. Yet, they consider this a state of remission and not a cure.

Let's look at another example. When someone has low back pain due to a pinched nerve and gets the problem resolved by seeing a chiropractor, is this person cured? Obviously this depends upon a number of different factors, such as what's causing the pinched nerve. But even if someone with a pinched nerve sees a chiropractor, receives treatment, and then it's determined that he or she is "cured", one can't argue that this person can suffer a "relapse" if they did the same things which originally caused the pinched nerve to develop in the first place. So if the pinched nerve was caused by lifting heavy objects on a frequent basis, combined with poor lifting techniques, there is a good chance the low back condition will "flare up" again if the person were to go back to this way of lifting.

What's The Difference Between A "Cure" And A "State Of Remission"?

When you think about it then, a cure really isn't much different than a state of remission. In fact, just about every condition which can be cured can return, although there are certain exceptions. Of course the word "cure" is used rather loosely. For example, many endocrinologists consider radioactive iodine treatment as being a "cure" for hyperthyroidism. I've even read material which states that RAI is a cure for these conditions, and then goes on to mention how the person will need to take thyroid hormone daily for the rest of their life after receiving radioactive iodine.

If you're talking about a permanent cure for the hyperthyroid symptoms then perhaps this is true. But this harsh treatment method is not curing the cause of the condition, as all it's doing is obliterating the thyroid gland in order to stop the excess production of thyroid hormone. So receiving radioactive iodine won't do anything for the underlying cause of the condition, as mentioned earlier in this book.

So do I consider my Graves' disease condition as being permanently cured? After all, it's been ten years since I wrote the second edition of this book, and while I've had some scares (i.e. chronic Lyme disease in 2018), I have been able to maintain a state of wellness since 2009. I'd like to think I'm cured, as if I were to visit an endocrinologist and didn't tell them that I was previously diagnosed with Graves' disease, and then went on to receive all of the standard testing (thyroid blood tests, tests for thyroid antibodies, etc.), I'm confident that all of these tests would come out negative, which means they wouldn't label me as having Graves' disease. But then again, these tests don't reveal what the underlying cause of the condition is, and what's happening on a cellular level. So even if I received all of these tests and they came out negative, this wouldn't necessarily mean that I was cured.

As a result, one needs to look into some of the other "alternative" tests I received. For example, one such test I did was an Adrenal Stress Index (ASI) test, which is a saliva test that measures the levels of cortisol, as well as some other hormones (DHEA, 17-hydroxyprogesterone, etc.). It also tests for the total salivary SIgA (also known as secretory IgA), which gives an indication of the health of both the gut and immune system. These tests did improve significantly after taking a natural treatment approach, as my depressed morning cortisol levels were within normal limits the last time I retested, and my DHEA also normalized after being depressed.

However, even if some of the values on the ASI test were abnormal, this still wouldn't confirm that I had Graves' disease. After all, many people who never have been diagnosed with Graves' disease have compromised adrenal glands, including low morning cortisol levels. Other people with Graves' disease have high cortisol levels. In other words, having high or low cortisol levels, a low DHEA, and/or a depressed total salivary SIgA doesn't confirm the presence or absence of hyperthyroidism. However, many people with hyperthyroid conditions do have imbalances in the cortisol levels, DHEA, and/or a depressed total salivary SIgA.

The same thing can be said with other "alternative" tests as well. Let's look at another example involving a woman who was diagnosed with Graves' disease and obtained a comprehensive stool panel, which revealed a lot of gut dysbiosis (imbalance of the gut flora), along with parasites. These factors can be contributing to her Graves' disease condition, but one can't definitively conclude this. In any case, if this woman were to take a natural treatment approach to restore her gut health and she eventually had no hyperthyroid symptoms, and if all of the conventional medical tests to diagnose Graves' disease were negative, but if she still had some gut imbalances upon retesting, could we still conclude that her Graves' disease condition was cured, in a state of remission, or neither one?

The problem is that while alternative tests such as an adrenal saliva test, dried urine test, hair mineral analysis test, comprehensive stool test, or organic acids test can help to determine some of the triggers and underlying imbalances of hyperthyroidism and Graves' disease, one can't conclude that positive findings on any of these tests is in fact causing this condition. This of course doesn't mean they aren't important, as they are extremely valuable tests which provide important information for anyone with hyperthyroidism who is looking to restore their health.

My overall point is that even though I sometimes use the word "cure" when talking about natural treatment methods, the truth is that there really is no way to determine whether someone is permanently cured, even if all conventional and alternative tests are negative. And if this is discouraging to you, hopefully reading the rest of this chapter (as well as the rest of this book) will convince you that it's still worth giving natural treatment methods a try.

A Relapse Is Always Possible

What you need to understand is that after taking a natural treatment approach, if you don't have any symptoms, if all of the conventional medical tests are negative, and if all of the functional medicine tests look great, this doesn't mean you're permanently cured. This doesn't just apply to hyperthyroidism and Graves' disease, but most other health conditions as well. For example, when I had my chiropractic practice in Concord, North Carolina, if a patient of mine had neck pain and then had their condition corrected through chiropractic adjustments, this doesn't mean the condition was permanently cured, as I eluded to earlier with the "pinched nerve" example.

If this patient with the neck pain went and did the same things which caused the neck condition to develop in the first place, there is an excellent chance the neck pain would return. Similarly, if someone developed a cyst on their wrist due to some type of repetitive activity, and then had the cyst removed surgically, another cyst might develop if they kept stressing out the wrist.

With hyperthyroidism, it seems that lifestyle factors play a huge role in the development of this condition, as I have already mentioned. Therefore, even if someone with a hyperthyroid condition has no symptoms and all negative tests, both medical and alternative in nature, this doesn't mean they can't suffer a relapse if they revert back to the same unhealthy lifestyle they had before they took a natural treatment approach.

So for example, if they ate plenty of refined foods and sugars, unhealthy oils, and did a poor job of handling their stress before being diagnosed with hyperthyroidism, and then upon taking a natural treatment approach they began eating well, improved their stress handling skills, and received the appropriate adrenal support, this definitely would help them with the recovery process. However, if after restoring their health they began eating junk food again and let stress get the best of them, a relapse would be likely to occur. It might take a few months, or even a few years before the condition returned, but there is an excellent chance this would happen.

Symptoms And Blood Tests Are Important, But...

While a person's symptoms and blood test results are important factors, the truth is that the body is very complex. As a result, just because someone is asymptomatic and all the tests are negative doesn't mean they don't have any health issues, whether it be a condition such as hyperthyroidism or something else. After all, a person's symptoms is frequently the last thing to develop, which means that when a person develops a condition such as hyperthyroidism or Graves' disease, it usually takes some time until any symptoms are present. And by the time the blood tests are positive, the condition is also fully developed.

This is why it's important to look at alternative tests. But as I just mentioned before, these tests aren't specific for any condition. For example, while there may be certain adrenal and nutrient imbalances someone with hyperthyroidism is more likely to have, everyone is different, and there can be other imbalances that need to be addressed.

Similarly, many, if not all people with Graves' disease have an increase in intestinal permeability (a leaky gut), but so do others who have different autoimmune conditions. So while alternative tests can be extremely valuable, there is no specific alternative test to confirm the presence or absence of hyperthyroidism.

Let's Aim For A "Permanent Remission"

Let's get back to the original question for this chapter, which is "do natural treatment methods really provide a permanent cure?" The truth is that I honestly don't know, and neither does any healthcare professional. While I'd like to consider my Graves' disease condition as being permanently cured, I believe that if I went back to the previous lifestyle habits I followed before I was initially diagnosed that there is a good chance a relapse would occur.

That being said, even if the best case scenario for someone who took a natural treatment approach involved them being in a permanent state of remission by maintaining a healthy lifestyle after restoring their health, then I'm guessing that most people would accept this. I know that as long as I am able to avoid receiving radioactive iodine treatment or thyroid surgery that I would be perfectly fine with this. So while I'd like to think that natural treatment methods can offer a permanent cure to hyperthyroidism, even a permanent state of remission would be fine with most people if it meant not having to rely on medication or having their thyroid gland obliterated.

Chapter Summary

- An effective natural treatment protocol should do more than just manage your symptoms.
- A cure really isn't much different than a state of remission, as most conditions which can be "cured" can return.
- In addition to the conventional thyroid blood tests, one should evaluate some of the "alternative" tests out there (adrenal saliva test, comprehensive stool panel, etc.)
- However, when these functional medicine tests are negative, this doesn't conclude whether someone is permanently cured
- With hyperthyroidism, lifestyle factors play a huge role in the development of this condition.
- Even if natural treatment methods don't provide a permanent cure, but can provide a permanent state of remission, I think most people would be fine with this.

For access to the book references and resources, visit
savemythyroid.com/hyperbooknotes

CHAPTER 7

The Immune System Component Of Graves' Disease

FOR THOSE PEOPLE with an autoimmune condition such as Graves' disease it is essential to address the immune system component. While many people think of Graves' disease as being a thyroid disorder, the truth is that this is an autoimmune condition which affects the thyroid gland. It puzzles me how most medical doctors neglect the immune system component, and focus primarily on the thyroid gland. After all, every endocrinologist and medical doctor knows that the immune system is compromised in Graves' disease, and using antithyroid medication to suppress the production of thyroid hormone, or radioactive iodine to obliterate the thyroid gland or removing the thyroid through surgery won't do anything to help improve the health of the immune system.

Studies show that people who have autoimmune conditions such as Graves' disease are more likely to develop other autoimmune conditions in the future.[10, 11] This includes Hashimoto's thyroiditis, Rheumatoid arthritis, systemic lupus erythematosus, Celiac disease, Addison's disease, type 1 diabetes mellitus, and other autoimmune conditions. Of these, rheumatoid arthritis was the most common coexisting autoimmune disorder.[10]

And when you think about it, this shouldn't be a surprise, as if most endocrinologists don't do anything to help improve the health of the immune system of their patients who have an autoimmune thyroid condition, then their immune system will of course remain in a compromised state, and they will therefore remain more susceptible to developing other autoimmune conditions. After all, the same factors which triggered Graves' disease can also trigger other autoimmune conditions. While genetics can play an important role in the development of one or more autoimmune conditions, it would seem obvious that if one doesn't do anything to remove the triggers while also improving the health of their immune system when someone is diagnosed with Graves' disease, then that person will have a greater chance of developing other autoimmune conditions in the future.

For example, when I was initially diagnosed with Graves' disease, the endocrinologist I consulted with recommended that I take methimazole, along with a beta blocker. And even though I didn't take the medication, I respected the fact that she didn't recommend that I treat my condition with radioactive iodine (which I of course would have rejected anyway). But besides recommending the prescription drugs, she didn't recommend anything else which could have helped improve the health of my immune system and thus prevent future autoimmune conditions from developing. Nothing was done to detect and then remove the triggers and underlying imbalances. While removing the trigger and then restoring the health of the compromised areas might not be a surefire method of preventing another autoimmune condition from developing, one can at least reduce their chances of developing such a condition by removing the triggers and then restoring the health of the immune system, along with other compromised areas of the body.

As you know, the goal of most medical doctors is to manage your symptoms, and not necessarily address the cause of your condition. And don't get me wrong, as symptomatic relief is important, and sometimes taking prescription medication is necessary. This is especially true with many cases of hyperthyroidism, as if a person has a very high heart rate, then they might need to take antithyroid medication and/or a beta blocker for awhile to help manage the symptoms.

Once again, medical doctors are trained to manage the symptoms, and so I understand their approach when they tell someone with a hyperthyroid condition to take antithyroid drugs and/or a beta blocker. But it's still very frustrating that they don't do anything to help the person improve the health of their immune system.

The Goal Should Be To Detect And Remove Any Immune System Triggers

Although genetic factors play a role in the development of thyroid and autoimmune thyroid conditions, some external factor usually triggers the genetics. So as I'll discuss later in this book, not everyone with the genes for an autoimmune condition such as Graves' disease will develop this condition. There are numerous factors which can trigger an autoimmune response, and obviously is it important to detect and then remove these triggers in order for someone to restore their health. But it's important to understand that many times, just removing the trigger won't be enough to restore someone's health, as usually the compromised areas of the body will need to be addressed.

In order to correct the immune system problem, you should be aware of some of the factors which can lead to it becoming compromised in the first place. And while there are a number of different factors which can lead to a compromised immune system, there are five primary ones which can play a major role. You'll notice that these are factors which are repeatedly brought up in this book, and the reason for this is because neglecting these factors will affect many areas of the body, including the endocrine system, digestive system, cardiovascular system, and yes, the immune system.

So here are the five primary factors which can lead to a compromised immune system:

1. **Chronic stress.** As I'll discuss in detail in the next chapter, many people deal with chronic stress, which our bodies were not designed to handle. This chronic stress can and usually will affect the immune system and adrenals. And while a competent natural healthcare professional will usually address these areas, it is just as important to help the person manage their stress in order to aid in their recovery. While the odds of completely eliminating the stress from your life are very slim, chances are you can do a much better job of coping with it, which will do wonders when trying to restore the health of your immune system.

2. **Poor nutrition.** Just as is the case with stress management, I can easily dedicate an entire book just talking about proper nutrition, and I did this in my book the Hyperthyroid Healing Diet, which will be released in the first quarter of 2024. In this book you're reading now I do have a separate chapter on the importance of diet and nutrition (Chapter 11). In any case, poor nutrition without question can compromise your immune system.

And while taking quality nutritional supplements and/or herbal remedies can definitely assist in restoring the health of your immune system, supplements are no substitute for eating well. Just about everyone diagnosed with hyperthyroidism needs to eat better, but in addition to eating well, most people will need to take some quality nutritional supplements so they can obtain the nutrients they aren't getting from their food. As you probably know, most people don't get all of the nutrients from the foods they eat, which is why everyone should at least take some basic nutritional supplements each day.

But it's not just nutritional deficiencies which affect the health of the immune system. Eating a poor diet and/or eating foods you're sensitive to can potentially lead to an increase in intestinal permeability (a leaky gut), which as I mentioned in an earlier chapter, is a factor in the development of an autoimmune condition. Eating poorly will also lead to blood sugar imbalances, which can lead to conditions such as insulin resistance, and this in turn can lead to problems with inflammation and also affect the health of the immune system.[12, 13] So it's not just about nutrient deficiencies.

3. **Sleep deprivation.** This of course can go either way, as sometimes a person has no problem obtaining quality sleep until they develop an autoimmune thyroid condition. Then once they have the autoimmune disorder they begin having sleeping difficulties. On the other hand, some people who are healthy will neglect their sleep for a period of months, or even years, which can eventually lead to numerous health problems. And there is evidence that sleep disturbances can be either a cause or a consequence of certain immune and autoimmune conditions.[14]

For example, some people who work a typical 8 to 5 shift will stay up late each night, and will end up averaging only 5 or 6 hours of quality sleep on a nightly basis. Over time, this can definitely have a negative impact on their immune system. On the other hand, people who work odd shifts which affect their sleep patterns can also be affected.

Then there are people with an entrepreneurial background who spend countless hours on their business, getting up early in the morning and going to sleep late. This routine, combined with the stress of owning one's business, will almost definitely have a negative impact on their immune system. This type of work ethic also applies to many people working in the corporate world, as many people spend sixty or more hours per week on their job, and end up neglecting their health.

4. **Environmental toxins.** Someone can eat well, get ample sleep, and do a great job of managing stress, yet can still end up with a compromised immune system if they are constantly being exposed to environmental toxins. Of course these days it's not a question of exposure, as everyone is consistently being exposed to toxins. Visit www.scorecard.org, and you can see how much air pollution is in your town. And even if the outdoor pollution isn't too bad, one needs to consider the impact of household products we bring into our home, as many of them contain harsh chemicals.

Numerous studies have shown that indoor air pollution can affect immune system health.[15, 16] The person who has a house located near a busy road with many cars passing by will be exposed to more toxins on a daily basis than someone who lives further away from a busy road. Smoking is clearly associated with a higher risk of developing Graves' disease.[17] But of course there are other types of environmental toxins as well.

Let's not forget about the impact of heavy metals, such as the mercury present in fish and dental amalgams. I know we tend to overlook these and other environmental toxins, but they can have a serious effect on our health. While it is impossible to avoid environmental toxins completely, most people can do a better job of reducing their exposure. I'll discuss this in Chapter 14.

5. **Infections.** Just as is the case with environmental toxins, certain pathogens can compromise the immune system, thus triggering an autoimmune response. These infections can have either a direct or indirect effect on

the immune system. For example, certain viruses such as Epstein Barr or hepatitis C can potentially trigger an autoimmune response.

Gut microbes such as H. pylori or Candida albicans can also affect the immune system, or they can cause an increase in intestinal permeability, which in turn can be a factor in autoimmunity. Other pathogens which can directly or indirectly cause or contribute to an autoimmune thyroid condition such as Graves' disease include Borrelia burgdorferi, Yersinia enterocolitica, and even parasites. I have dedicated a separate chapter which discusses the relationship between infections and Graves' disease (Chapter 15).

Is The Immune System Weak Or Is It Overactive?

With regards to Graves' disease, I frequently talk about a "compromised" immune system, but what exactly does this mean? Does it mean the immune system is in a weakened state? Or does it refer to an overactive state? In a way it's a combination of both, although either way, the goal of an effective natural treatment protocol involves suppressing the autoimmune component and eliminating the inflammation which in turn will help improve the health of the immune system.

To clarify this, if someone has certain deficiencies, such as low Vitamin D and/or selenium levels, this can essentially "weaken" the immune system by causing a decrease in regulatory T cells. On the other hand, if this person also has high thyroid antibodies, which is characteristic of Graves' disease, then this would be considered to be an overactive state, which relates to an increase in Th17 cells. So in this example, one of the goals of a natural treatment approach would be to increase the Vitamin D and selenium levels to improve the health of the immune system by increasing the regulatory T cells, which in turn can help suppress the autoimmune component and lower the thyroid antibodies by decreasing Th17 cells.

In summary, if you have been diagnosed with an autoimmune thyroid condition, make sure you do what is necessary to restore the health of your immune system. You can of course try speaking with your endocrinologist or general medical practitioner about how to go about doing this, but as you know, most medical doctors don't receive adequate training in preventative care, which is why you'll see me constantly recommend for people with these conditions to speak with a competent natural healthcare professional. Because if you don't address the immune system component of Graves' disease, then it won't be possible to restore your health.

Chapter Summary

- For people with Graves' Disease, it's important to focus on improving the health of the immune system component.
- Research has shown that people who have autoimmune conditions such as Graves' disease are more likely to develop additional autoimmune conditions in the future, such as rheumatoid arthritis and Lupus.
- While it can be important to take antithyroid drugs, they do nothing for the compromised immune system.
- Five factors which can lead to a compromised immune system include: 1) chronic stress, 2) poor nutrition, 3) sleep deprivation, 4) environmental toxins, and 5) infections

For access to the book references and resources, visit
savemythyroid.com/hyperbooknotes

CHAPTER 8

The Role That Stress Plays In The Development Of Hyperthyroidism

As I BRIEFLY MENTIONED earlier in this book, stress can play a role in the development of hyperthyroidism. This is especially true with Graves' disease, although it can be a factor with other hyperthyroid conditions. I spoke about how chronic stress can negatively affect the adrenal glands, and in this chapter I'm going to go into greater detail about this.

I believe that chronic stress was a big factor in the development of my Graves' disease condition. Although I'm sure there were other factors as well, I definitely dealt with a lot of chronic stress for many years. Obviously a lot of people deal with chronic stress, and it's not just the stress itself which is the culprit, but it's the person's ability to handle the stress which is a big factor. And I admittedly didn't do a good job of managing my stress.

First of all it's important to understand that the human body wasn't designed to handle chronic stress. The adrenal glands were designed to handle acute stress situations without much of a problem. But in today's world most people are overwhelmed with chronic stress, as they have stressful jobs, stressful relationships, financial problems, and many other stressful issues. And even though stress is common, most people don't do a good job of managing the stress in their life, as I just mentioned before.

Since the adrenal glands weren't designed to handle chronic stress situations, for a person who deals with a lot of stress AND does a poor job of managing it, what frequently happens is over a period of months and years there is an excellent chance they will develop dysregulation of the hypothalamic pituitary adrenal (HPA) axis. Essentially they will have compromised adrenals, but the reason it's called HPA axis dysregulation is because the hypothalamus communicates with the pituitary gland, which in turn communicates with the adrenals.

How Stressed Out Adrenal Glands Can Affect The Thyroid Gland

There are a few different ways in which compromised adrenals can affect the thyroid gland. While high cortisol can have a negative effect on the conversion of T4 to T3, the focus here will be on the impact of stress on the immune system. Donna Jackson Nakazawa, who is the author of the book "The Autoimmune Epidemic", reveals how high cortisol levels affects immunity:

> *"Prolonged levels of heightened cortisol can not only lead to an underfunctioning immune system, but can also indirectly stimulate an autoimmune response. Cortisol helps to regulate our immune-system response not only by turning on the immune response, but also by turning it off. When cortisol keeps being pumped out because of daily anxieties and stressors, we stop*

producing sufficient cortisol to signal the immune response to turn off. This increases the likelihood that the immune system will go into erratic overdrive, that mistakes will be made and autoantibodies will attack the body itself".[18]

But what about depressed cortisol levels? Some people with hyperthyroidism have elevated cortisol levels, while others have depressed cortisol levels. The latter situation described myself, as I had depressed cortisol levels when I was diagnosed with Graves' disease. To better understand the process let's look at what Dr. James Wilson, author of the well know book "Adrenal Fatigue" has to say about how the adrenal glands affect the immune system:

"When cortisol is elevated during an alarm reaction, there is almost a complete disappearance of lymphocytes from the blood. That is why your immune system is suppressed when you are under stress or taking corticosteroids. On the other hand when circulating cortisol is low, its moderating effect on immune reactions is lost and lymphocytes circulate in excess. In this situation inflammation is greater with more redness and swelling, and it takes a longer time for the inflamed tissue to return to normal. So, directly and indirectly cortisol dramatically influences most aspects of immune function".[19]

To explain this in a different way, whether someone has high or low cortisol levels they will have dysregulation of the HPA axis, which can cause a proinflammatory state, and this in turn can lead to the development of an autoimmune condition. You don't want cortisol to be too high, but you also need sufficient cortisol to help regulate inflammation. So if cortisol is too high or low it can result in a proinflammatory state.

I should also mention that chronic stress can result in a decrease in secretory IgA, which lines the mucosal surfaces of the body, including the gastrointestinal tract. And if someone has lower secretory IgA they will be more prone to developing food sensitivities and infections, both of which can be potential triggers of Graves' disease. It's also worth mentioning that many people with a low secretory IgA won't experience digestive symptoms, which is one reason why the lack of digestive symptoms doesn't rule out gut problems.

What Does The Research Show?

There are a few different studies showing a relationship between stress and Graves' disease. One study of people with Graves' disease suggested that major life events was a factor in the development of a hyperthyroid condition, and that "coping strategies" may help to improve the prognosis in people with Graves' disease.[20] This study didn't conclude that stress was the main cause of Graves' disease, and I'm definitely not suggesting that stress is the primary cause of this or any other hyperthyroid condition, but I think there's little doubt that stress can play a huge role in the development of these conditions. Numerous other studies also have shown a correlation between stressful life events and Graves' disease.[21, 22]

Most Medical Doctors Don't Do Anything To Improve Adrenal Health

In the previous chapter I discussed how most medical doctors don't do anything to address the immune system component of Graves' disease. This is true even though every endocrinologist and medical doctor knows that Graves' disease is an autoimmune condition. So it shouldn't surprise you that most endocrinologists don't do anything to improve the health of the adrenals either.

Because in order to do this they would first need to determine whether someone has compromised adrenal glands to begin with, which they almost never do. There are exceptions, as if they suspect a person has a severe condition such as Addison's disease or Cushing's syndrome, then they will take a look at their morning cortisol, ACTH, and perhaps run some other tests. But even though many people have adrenal imbalances as a result of HPA axis dysregulation, most medical doctors usually don't do anything to evaluate this, let alone treat it. And once again, this is due to the training they receive in medical school.

My goal here isn't to bash the medical profession. I just want to make you aware of this, so that you can understand yet another difference between visiting an endocrinologist and seeing a natural healthcare practitioner.

It's Not Just About Emotional Stressors

I should add that it wasn't just about emotional stress in my situation, as while this definitely was a factor, I was also overtraining prior to my Graves' disease diagnosis. While I encourage people to be active and to exercise regularly, excess exercise can also disrupt the HPA axis and lead to adrenal imbalances. With my background I should have known better at the time, but I'm sharing this because over the years I've worked with people who also were exercising excessively before being diagnosed with hyperthyroidism.

How To Determine Whether Someone Has HPA Axis Dysregulation

One of the best methods of determining whether someone has compromised adrenal glands is through saliva testing. There are numerous companies which offer such testing, and most of them involve the person collecting four saliva samples at different intervals throughout the day, which correlate with the circadian pattern. This is far more valuable than a single cortisol sample, which is what most medical doctors will recommend. Most medical doctors will recommend a single serum cortisol sample in the morning, and if it's depressed or elevated, they will determine that the person has a problem with their adrenal glands. This might be true, but it's best to look at the cortisol levels throughout the day.

I should also mention that when I give recommendations based on the results of adrenal testing, there will be differences in the protocol for someone who has high cortisol levels when compared to someone who has depressed cortisol levels. For example, if someone has depressed cortisol levels I will frequently recommend the herb licorice (as long as they don't have high blood pressure), but I typically recommend different natural agents for someone who has high cortisol levels. And I've consulted with many patients who had normal or low cortisol levels in the morning, but had high cortisol levels later in the day. So once again, just obtaining a one sample cortisol test in the morning isn't sufficient.

If you're concerned about the accuracy of saliva testing, numerous studies have shown that saliva testing is just as accurate as serum testing when it comes to looking at the cortisol levels.[23, 24, 25] In fact, one study suggests that salivary cortisol is a more appropriate testing measure for the clinical assessment of adrenocortical function than serum cortisol.[26] One thing to keep in mind is that cortisol rises in response to stress, and many people become stressed out when visiting the doctor and/or upon the injection they receive when drawing the blood.

And so this potentially can result in a false elevation of the serum cortisol levels. This can also happen with saliva testing, as for example, if you were to have a stressful morning when collecting the first saliva sample this can result in cortisol being elevated when it normally wouldn't be. As a result, if stress is normally high then it's fine to collect the saliva samples on that day, but I wouldn't collect the saliva samples if your stress is abnormally high, and if you start collecting them and have an abnormally stressful day you might want to consider recollecting the samples.

A Breakdown of The Adrenal Saliva Test

Let's take a look at what the adrenal saliva test I use measures. Please keep in mind that different labs will look at different markers, but the main commonality is that they will test the cortisol levels throughout the day, which means you will be collecting multiple saliva samples, starting in the morning, and then the last one is usually before going to bed.

Cortisol levels: This is the primary hormone most natural healthcare practitioners will look at on this test, as this test will measure four different cortisol levels throughout the day to determine if you have a proper circadian pattern. Normally the cortisol levels should be at the highest levels in the morning upon waking up, and will decrease throughout the day. This pattern will help to give you the energy you need throughout the day, and the lower cortisol levels at night will allow you to fall asleep. These patterns will differ for someone who works odd or alternating shifts.

So increased cortisol levels are more common in the beginning phases of adrenal imbalances. In other words, when someone does something to stress out their adrenals on a chronic basis, whether it's eat a lot of refined foods and sugars, get insufficient sleep, or do a poor job of managing their stress, initially the adrenals will do a good job of compensating. And so for many months, or in some cases for many years, the adrenals will secrete either normal or higher amounts of cortisol. But over time what commonly happens it that the adrenals will lose the ability to adapt to the chronic stress, and therefore will secrete less and less cortisol, until these levels become depressed.

DHEA/DHEA-S: DHEA is manufactured by the adrenal glands, and it plays a big role in immunity and in the stress response. DHEAS is the sulfated version of DHEA. As you know by now, if someone deals with chronic stress on a regular basis, this will lead to HPA axis dysregulation, and this can also affect the DHEA levels, causing them to become low over time. But just as is the case with cortisol, in the beginning phases the body will usually do a good job of compensating, and so it's common to see the DHEA normal even when someone has compromised adrenal glands. On a saliva test it might initially present as high cortisol and normal DHEA.

17-OH Progesterone: A steroid hormone that is a precursor to cortisol, and is produced during the synthesis of glucocorticoids and sex steroids. This hormone is mainly produced in the adrenal glands, and when someone has compromised adrenals these hormone levels will commonly be less than optimal. Keep in mind that this isn't exactly the same as progesterone, but since they share the same biochemical pathway, if someone has a low 17-OH progesterone then there is a good chance that they also have low progesterone levels.

Secretory IgA: I mentioned this earlier, as this is an antibody found in the mucosal surfaces which plays an important role in immunity. SIgA is produced by B-cells in the mucosa, and it forms immune complexes with pathogens (i.e. viruses, bacteria), and therefore helps to protect the GI tract. Low values can indicate a problem with both the gut and immune system. And when someone has depressed SIgA levels, this makes them more susceptible to infections, food sensitivities, and even autoimmune conditions.

People with depressed SIgA levels are more likely to have an increased intestinal permeability and gut dysbiosis. And not everyone who has depressed levels of SIgA experiences symptoms. I do need to mention that not all saliva companies include secretory IgA as a marker, and some comprehensive stool panels include this marker as well.

How about elevated SIgA levels? When someone has elevated SIgA levels this means that there is some type of immune reaction. Usually it's a result of a food sensitivity or infection. And so it might take some detective work to determine why the levels are elevated.

Gliadin antibodies: Elevated gliadin antibodies indicate an immune response to gluten. Consuming gluten can cause a lot of problems whether someone has a gluten sensitivity or not, which is why I'm not a big fan of the lab including this marker on their adrenal saliva test. While an elevated level will make someone aware that they have a gluten sensitivity, if someone has a negative finding then they might conclude that it's fine to eat gluten, not realizing that even if someone doesn't have a gluten sensitivity that it can still increase the permeability of the gut.

It's also important to mention that this test may not be completely accurate in someone with a depressed secretory IgA. Also, if someone has been on a gluten free diet for a few months then we would expect this to be negative. Finally, alpha-gliadin is only one of the proteins of gluten, as with a Celiac panel they look at other factors which may indicate that someone reacts to gluten, such as evaluating transglutaminase and the endomysial antibodies. As a result, I don't rely on testing for the gliadin antibodies alone to determine if someone has an issue with gluten.

For my patients I recommend either a Celiac Panel, or another option is the Wheat/Gluten Proteome Reactivity & Autoimmunity test by the company Cyrex Labs, which a comprehensive test for gluten. This tests for the IgG and IgA antibodies against the proteins, peptides, and certain enzymes associated with a gluten sensitivity. I usually don't recommend this test, as if someone is eating gluten I'll recommend a Celiac panel, as Celiac disease is much more common in those with

Graves' disease[27, 28]. But even if they don't have Celiac disease I'll recommend for them to avoid gluten while trying to heal, which I'll discuss more in Chapter 11.

Saliva vs. Dried Urine Testing

Although I've been using saliva testing as a way of evaluating adrenal health since 2009, in 2017 I started using dried urine testing on some of my patients. Like saliva testing, dried urine testing also looks at the circadian rhythm of cortisol, as it involves collecting multiple samples throughout the day. If you're just focusing on the adrenals I think saliva testing is fine, but if you also want a comprehensive test that looks at the sex hormones (i.e. estrogen, progesterone), along with the metabolism of the hormones, then you might want to consider dried urine testing.

Of course you can always test the sex hormones through the blood, but the urine is the only place where you can look at the metabolism of some of the hormones. Estrogen is the main one to look at, as problems with estrogen metabolism can be a factor in the development of thyroid nodules, along with uterine fibroids, ovarian cysts, and endometriosis. Another reason to look at the estrogen metabolites is if there is a personal or family history of estrogen-dependent cancer.

How Can You Tell If You Would Benefit From Adrenal Testing?

If you're consulting with a competent natural healthcare practitioner, they will have you complete a comprehensive health history which can help determine if you might have adrenal imbalances. Some of the more common symptoms include fatigue, sugar cravings, and sleep disturbances, although there are numerous other symptoms one can have. Of course other factors can cause similar symptoms, and so there are times when additional testing might be necessary to obtain.

And you can't go by symptoms alone, as when I was diagnosed with Graves' disease both my cortisol levels and DHEA were depressed, which commonly result in fatigue, but I felt fine from an energy standpoint, and I didn't have any sleep issues. While I don't recommend self-treating the adrenals, upon being diagnosed by a competent natural healthcare professional you can do some things on your own to assist in your recovery. Probably the most important thing you can do is work on improving your stress handling skills.

For those who are unable to afford saliva testing or dried urine testing, if you read the book "Adrenal Fatigue, the 21st Century Syndrome" by Dr. James Wilson, he includes some detailed questionnaires to help determine if you have problems with your adrenal glands. While you can't rely on symptoms alone, I do think the questionnaires have some value and are worth checking out.

You can find another excellent adrenal assessment in the book "The Adrenal Transformation Protocol". This was written by my friend Dr. Izabella Wentz, who has three amazing books on Hashimoto's thyroiditis, and I can't say enough about her more recent book that focuses on the adrenals.

How To Restore The Health Of The Adrenals

In order to restore the health of the adrenal glands, one obviously needs to address the cause of the problem. With regards to stress, it is just about impossible to eliminate all of the stress from your life. On the other hand, there are two things you can do when it comes to dealing with chronic stress which will lead to better health:

1. **Minimize the number of stressful situations.** Once again, you won't be able to eliminate all of the stress in your life, but in many cases it is possible to reduce some of the stressful situations you are dealing with.

Write down all of the different things in your life that you consider to be stressful, and try to figure out how you can make some changes to make things less stressful.

2. **Learn how to better cope with the stress in your life.** While it might be difficult to eliminate some of the stressful situations in your life, you do need to learn how to do a good job of managing stress. Of course there are many different ways to manage stress, as one can exercise or do yoga, get a relaxation massage every now and then, have a counseling session, eat a healthier diet, get more sleep each night, etc. These obviously are just a handful of basic examples, but I think you get the picture.

Biofeedback is a technique many people can benefit from to help them better manage the stress in their life. I use a program called HeartMath, which measures heart rate variability. For more information I'd recommend visiting the website www.heartmath.com. The device I have is called the Inner Balance, which is compatible with your smart phone, although they also have an option if you prefer installing the program on a computer.

If you deal with a great amount of stress and are willing to block out a small amount of time each day to use this program then it can be well worth the investment. On the other hand, if you don't use the program on a frequent basis then it probably would be best not to get it. I will say that most of my patients don't invest in HeartMath, as most incorporate mind body medicine techniques such as yoga, meditation, or simply deep breathing.

12 Stress Management Tips You Can Follow

In a previous article on my website I discussed twelve stress management tips to help restore someone's thyroid health, and included this in the second edition of the book. I've gone ahead and updated these tips, and figured it would be a good idea to include them here in this updated third edition:

Tip #1: Try to keep a positive attitude most of the time. While a positive attitude alone isn't enough to manage your stress, keeping positive can definitely help. Obviously nobody can be positive 100% of the time. But many people seem to always carry a negative attitude with them, which definitely won't help you cope with the stress in your life.

Tip #2: Block out at least five minutes per day for stress management. The goal here is to get into the daily routine of stress management. I recommend to start with five minutes per day, and then you can gradually increase the duration until you are blocking out 10-15 minutes on some days, and perhaps even longer on some days.

Tip #3: Aim for eight hours of sleep each night. Admittedly there are some people who don't need eight hours of sleep, and I personally think I do fine with 7 ½ hours of sleep. But there is no denying that getting sufficient sleep is important for healthy adrenals, which in turn will help improve your stress handling skills. And assuming it takes some time for you to fall asleep you'll need to account for this. So for example, if you're aiming for eight hours sleep and on average it takes you fifteen minutes to fall asleep then you'll want to be in bed for eight hours and fifteen minutes.

Tip #4: Eat healthier foods. Most of us can do a much better job of incorporating healthier foods into our diets, which also can have positive benefits on the adrenals. I don't expect anyone who has been eating poorly to immediately give up all of the "bad foods" they love. But even making small changes in what you eat can have a big impact on your health, and then hopefully over time you'll make even more positive changes when it comes to what you eat. That being said, if you want to make more abrupt changes to your diet that's perfectly fine. I will discuss diet in greater detail in Chapter 11.

Tip #5: Exercise regularly, but not excessively. It's important to be active on a daily basis, although with hyperthyroidism you do want to be cautious, as many people already have an elevated resting heart rate, and you don't want it to get too high. But regular exercise can also help you to better manage stress, and in addition to some light cardiovascular exercise on a daily basis, I would also recommend to do some resistance training three to four times per week. Of course if you haven't exercised for awhile you do need to start out slow, and it's also wise to consult with your medical doctor first.

Tip #6: Keep a daily gratitude journal. Keeping a daily gratitude journal is another way to help manage your stress better. When I dealt with Graves' disease it was definitely very stressful, but I still had a lot to be grateful for. But sometimes we focus on the negative, and so it helps to put in writing what we're grateful for, and this is something that shouldn't take more than a few minutes each day.

Tip #7: Take nutritional supplements and herbs. Certain nutritional supplements and herbs can help us to better manage the stress in our life. And I'm not just talking about specific supplements that can support the adrenals , but even some common deficiencies can make it more challenging to cope with the stress. Examples include deficiencies in omega-3 fatty acids and vitamin D. I'll talk more about nutritional supplements in Chapter 12.

Tip #8: Consider acupuncture. There are a lot of different health benefits of acupuncture, and research shows that it can also serve as a form of stress management.[29, 30]

Tip #9: Get a monthly massage. Schedule an appointment with a licensed massage therapist and treat yourself to a monthly massage. Massage therapy is not just about stress management, as it can help to increase lymphatic flow, help to decrease muscular pain and spasms, and there are many other benefits as well. But one of the big benefits of massage therapy is that it can help to relieve stress.

Tip #10: Consider seeing a chiropractor. Okay, I'm admittedly a little bit biased here, being that I have a chiropractic background. But since spinal adjustments help to balance out the nervous system, receiving them from a chiropractor can also help to relieve stress. Like massage therapy, there are so many other benefits when it comes to chiropractic.

Tip #11: Talk to someone. Sometimes speaking with someone can help relieve your stress. This doesn't necessarily mean talking with a counselor, although in some cases this can be helpful. But even talking with a good friend, family member, or acquaintance can help.

Tip #12: Don't take life so seriously. This doesn't mean that you shouldn't take certain aspects of your life seriously. But on the other hand, many of us let things stress us out that really shouldn't. Write down a list of some of the things which cause stress in your life, and then take a look at these tips I have just given you, and determine how you can apply this advice to those things that stress you out on a regular basis.

For example, if you have a job that stresses you out, then perhaps you need to change your attitude (or change your job!). Or it might be that you're not eating well and/or not getting enough sleep. These lifestyle changes won't eliminate the stress in your life, but will help you to better manage it. If your spouse is stressing you out, then perhaps counseling is the answer for you.

So here you have it, as if you follow at least 75% of these tips, including the first six I listed, you will do wonders in managing your stress. This admittedly is an incomplete list, as there are other things you can do to manage your stress. But these are some of the more important ones that can truly help to restore your health, and help you to maintain your health.

High Energy Levels Don't Equal Healthy Adrenals

I just wanted to remind you that just because someone has compromised adrenals doesn't mean they will have low energy levels. Although having low energy levels is very common, some people with hyperthyroidism have adrenal imbalances, yet have high energy levels. As I mentioned earlier in this chapter, I personally felt great from an energy standpoint after being diagnosed with hyperthyroidism, yet the adrenal saliva test showed that I had depressed cortisol levels, along with a depressed DHEA. Over the years I have consulted with many other people with hyperthyroidism who also had a lot of energy months after being diagnosed, and didn't feel fatigued, even though their saliva test revealed imbalances of their adrenal glands.

It once again is important to understand that it usually takes a good amount of time for the adrenal glands to become compromised. And once they become compromised, it then usually takes time for a person to become symptomatic. Some people develop fatigue quicker than others, but eventually most people with adrenal imbalances will develop lower energy levels. So you can't rely on symptoms alone, and therefore we can't assume that someone who has high energy levels has perfectly healthy adrenal glands.

In summary, chronic stress can cause a lot of different problems, and if not managed effectively it will affect the adrenal glands, which in turn can ultimately cause or contribute to hyperthyroidism. Of course this doesn't mean that all hyperthyroid conditions are caused by stress, but there's no question that stress is a factor in many cases. And for those who have a hyperthyroid condition which was caused by stress, doing a better job of managing the stress in their life is essential if they want to use natural thyroid treatment methods to restore their health. But even for those who choose conventional medical treatments, it still will benefit your overall health to become an expert in stress management.

Chapter Summary

- Prolonged stress and adrenal imbalances can be a big factor in the development of hyperthyroidism.
- An adrenal saliva test can help determine whether someone has a problem with their adrenals.
- Dried urine testing is another option to help determine whether someone has adrenal imbalances.
- In order to restore the health of the adrenal glands, one needs to determine what caused the problem with their adrenal glands in the first place.
- Reading the 12 stress management tips listed in this chapter will help you to better manage your stress, which in turn will help improve your adrenal health.

For access to the book references and resources, visit
savemythyroid.com/hyperbooknotes

CHAPTER 9

The Importance Of Proper Digestion In Restoring Your Health

I ENJOYED WORKING with Roy to help him address his Graves' disease condition. And while he was showing progress, his thyroid stimulating immunoglobulins wouldn't decrease any further. Although I was thinking about recommending a comprehensive stool panel, I didn't think it would show anything since he didn't experience any digestive symptoms, had regular bowel movements, etc.

Even though this took place many years ago and only a few years after I started helping people with thyroid and autoimmune thyroid conditions, I still should have known better than to rely on Roy's lack of symptoms. In other words, the lack of digestive symptoms doesn't rule out a gut problem. But back then I told Roy that I didn't think a comprehensive stool test would reveal anything significant, and therefore didn't recommend one to him.

Roy stopped seeing me, and I decided to follow-up with him approximately six months later. He told me that he ended up seeing another natural healthcare practitioner, who did do a comprehensive stool panel, and Roy tested positive for parasites. To make a long story short, the natural healthcare practitioner gave Roy recommendations, which in turn eradicated the parasites, and Roy's thyroid stimulating immunoglobulins normalized.

I wouldn't have found this out had I not followed up with Roy, but I'm glad I did, as it taught me a valuable lesson. I'm not telling this story to suggest that everyone reading this book should do a comprehensive stool panel, and I can't say that I recommend one to all of my patients. But if I don't recommend a stool test initially and the person isn't progressing, I won't hesitate to recommend one, even if the person's gut health seems to be fine.

Don't Overlook The Importance Of Having A Healthy Gut Microbiome

When it comes to restoring one's health after being diagnosed with hyperthyroidism, one of the most important factors is how well you digest and absorb your food. In the next few chapters I will focus a great deal on eating well and the importance of proper nutritional supplementation. In fact, if you read any book that focuses on natural treatment methods for a specific condition, chances are it will discuss in detail how you need to eat well, and many will also talk about nutritional supplementation.

However, eating quality foods and taking nutritional supplements won't do you much good if you aren't properly digesting and absorbing what you consume. Many people's digestive systems are not functioning properly, and so their body does a poor job of digesting and absorbing the food they eat and the supplements they take, which means they won't receive optimal benefits from them. This is yet another reason why someone who has been eating junk food on a daily basis for many years usually can't get well simply by changing their diet and taking supplements.

Many People Have An Increase In Intestinal Permeability

A lot of people have an increase in intestinal permeability, which is the medical term for a "leaky gut". I briefly mentioned this in Chapter 4, and I'll discuss this condition in greater detail in Chapter 10. But what's important to understand is that there are many different factors which can lead to a leaky gut, and so in order to heal the gut these factors need to be removed. Taking digestive enzymes, probiotics, and drinking bone broth and supplementing with L-glutamine can also help with gut healing, as can other factors, but you absolutely need to remove anything that is causing the leaky gut.

Although I used to frequently test my patients to determine if they have a leaky gut, these days I just assume that the people I work with have this condition. And the reason for this is because when I regularly did leaky gut testing in the past, most people tested positive. In addition, for those who have Graves' disease, there is something called the "Triad of Autoimmunity", which says that there are three factors necessary for autoimmunity to develop. This includes a genetic predisposition, exposure to one or more environmental triggers, and an increase in intestinal permeability.

While there is nothing you can do from a genetic predisposition stand-point, you can find and remove the environmental triggers, and do things to heal the gut.

The Dangers Of Acid-Blocking Medication

While most people are aware of the negative impact of antibiotics on the gut microbiome, millions of people take acid-blocking medication, which arguably is just as bad, and can have a lot of negative consequences. Let's just think about this for a minute. One needs a good amount of acid in their stomach to digest the food they eat and any minerals they take. So if you take drugs which reduce the production of gastric acid then there is no way you can properly digest the food and supplemental minerals you ingest.

Of course if you have an excessive amount of stomach acid then perhaps these drugs can help (although they won't get to the underlying cause of the problem). But many people are told to take acid-blocking medication based solely on the symptoms they are experiencing, without confirming whether or not they truly have an excessive amount of stomach acid being produced. It's also important to mention that gastric acid not only is important when it comes to the digestive process, but also plays a role in keeping bacteria and yeast in check. And so a deficiency in stomach acid can lead to conditions such as yeast overgrowth and/or SIBO (small intestinal bacterial overgrowth).

Is it wise to take acid-blocking medication if you experience a lot of stomach burning and/or acid reflux? This isn't always related to an increase in the amount of stomach acid, as it can be caused by a decrease in the lining of your stomach due to poor eating habits, increased stress, and other lifestyle factors. And even when such symptoms are caused by an increase in stomach acid, the goal still should be to get to the cause of the problem. So yes, if you have high stomach acid levels then taking acid-blocking medication may help to manage the symptoms, but it will do absolutely nothing for the underlying cause of the problem. And the long term side effects it can have on your digestive system, your bone density, and other areas of your body can be disastrous.

Healing The Gut Can Take Awhile

Depending on the cause of the digestive issues, it can take a good amount of time to heal. Eating well is always a good place to start when trying to restore one's gut health, although doing this alone isn't always the answer. I realize that many people reading this book have already made some great changes to their diet, which is fantastic. But in many cases there is still room for improvement, and going beyond diet is frequently necessary.

When trying to restore the health of the gut microbiome, a person might benefit from taking certain nutritional supplements, including prebiotics, probiotics, and digestive enzymes. In many cases it can also be beneficial to take betaine HCL or bitter herbs if someone has low stomach acid, which is common, and sometimes bile salts can also provide some great benefits. I'll talk more about supplements in Chapter 12, and while I currently take prebiotics and probiotic supplements on a wellness basis, most people shouldn't have to rely on taking digestive enzymes on a permanent basis.

7 Tips To Help Improve Your Digestive Health

What I'd like to do now is discuss seven different things you can do in order to improve your digestive health. Most of these you can do immediately, and while they might require some dramatic changes in your current lifestyle, I can almost guarantee you will feel much better than you currently do after incorporating some or all these changes. So let's take a look at how you can improve your digestion:

Healthy Digestion Tip #1: Avoid eating common food allergens. The main common food allergens I'll mention here are gluten, dairy, corn, and soy, with arguably the first three being the most important to avoid while restoring your health. A lot of practitioners focus on avoiding gluten, but corn can be just as problematic for many people, and therefore should be eliminated while trying to heal the gut.

Healthy Digestion Tip #2: Avoid other foods that can be harsh on the gut. In addition to avoiding common food allergens, to assist with healing your gut I would also try your best to avoid nightshades (tomatoes, eggplant, peppers, white potatoes), grains, and legumes. I discuss this more in Chapter 11, and I know this will be met with a lot of resistance, and ultimately it's up to you as to whether you avoid them or continue to eat them. If you happen to be a vegan or vegetarian I understand that it probably will be challenging to completely eliminate grains and legumes from your diet. Once again, I'll discuss this in Chapter 11.

Just keep in mind that I'm not suggesting that you should permanently avoid nightshades, grains, and legumes, as most people can eventually reintroduce them. But there is a reason why these foods are excluded on an autoimmune protocol (also discussed in Chapter 11), and why grains and legumes are not part of a standard Paleo diet either. All three of these categories of foods have compounds which can have a negative effect on gut healing.

Healthy Digestion Tip #3: Address any gut infections. If you have a bacterial, yeast, or parasitic infection affecting the gut then you'll want to address this. Even though yeast/fungal infections do happen, in most cases people actually experience a yeast overgrowth, and not a true infection. However, a yeast overgrowth can have a negative effect on the intestinal barrier, and so can small intestinal bacterial overgrowth (SIBO). And so when I say "gut infections" I'm mainly referring to bacteria such as H. pylori and yersinia enterocolitica, as well as parasites.

I already spoke about H. pylori in Chapter 4, but I want to add that there is controversy over the pathogenicity of H. pylori and parasites.

In other words, some healthcare practitioners feel like both H. pylori and certain parasites (i.e. Blastocystis Hominis) are commensal (part of the normal gut flora), and therefore shouldn't be eradicated. I think it depends on the situation, as I don't think that healthy individuals should be doing parasite cleanses on a regular basis, and I also agree that H. pylori isn't always harmful.

But for many years I've been putting those with Graves' disease on what I consider to be a more gentle protocol when H. pylori is detected. And I admit that I also will treat some people for parasites using an herbal approach. On the other hand, I do think that most people with H. pylori and parasites don't need to take prescription drugs (i.e. antibiotics). While there is a time and place for antibiotics, since they disrupt the gut microbiome you shouldn't take them unless if absolutely necessary.

Healthy Digestion Tip #4: Consider taking digestive enzymes, betaine HCL, and/or bile salts. I already mentioned this, and in many cases I give my patients a supplement called Enzymes Plus that has all three of these, although there are times when someone might need to take additional betaine HCL and/or bile salts. And once again, the goal isn't to be on these permanently.

Healthy Digestion Tip #5: Increase your fiber intake. Most people don't consume enough fiber, which is a big reason why many people are constipated (although it's certainly not the only reason). And while I experienced chronic constipation as a teenager and young adult, I realize that a lot of people with hyperthyroidism experience the opposite problem. In other words, many people with hyperthyroidism experience an excessive amount of bowel movements per day. Arguably it's better to have four or five bowel movements per day than one bowel movement every few days.

But fiber isn't just about supporting regular bowel movements, as it also is beneficial for the gut microbiome. About 20 to 35 grams of fiber is needed per day,[31] and most people are lucky to consume half this amount with the way they eat. You can ensure you get enough fiber by eating plenty of fruits and vegetables, especially fiber-rich fruit and vegetables such as apples, artichokes, asparagus, broccoli, pears, and sweet potatoes.

Assuming someone isn't on an AIP diet then they can eat nuts, which also can be a good source of fiber. But even if you rely on fruits and vegetables it's very possible to get enough fiber. I will admit that there are some situations where eating more fiber can result in bloating, gas, and sometimes even constipation. This isn't the norm, but when it does happen I would suspect a problem such as small intestinal bacterial overgrowth (SIBO).

During the healing process I would make sure to listen to your body, as if you experience digestive symptoms when eating high-fiber foods then you might need to temporarily cut back. Similarly, if you have problems with raw vegetables but are able to tolerate them when they're cooked, then focus on eating cooked vegetables while trying to restore the health of the gut microbiome.

Healthy Digestion Tip #6: Incorporate gut healing foods and supplements.
Drinking bone broth and eating fermented foods such as sauerkraut can help to support the healing of the gut. This doesn't mean that you need to consume these to heal your gut, but doing so can help to accelerate the process. Similarly, certain nutritional supplements and herbs can assist in gut healing, which I'll talk more about in Chapter 10.

Healthy Digestion Tip #7: Improve your stress handling skills. Since stress can have a negative impact on the gut, this is yet another reason to improve your stress handling skills. I already discussed this in Chapter 8, but I wanted to bring it up here, because even if you eat an extremely healthy diet, but are stressed out all of the time, this can prevent your gut from healing.

So there you go! Seven things you can and should do in order to ensure a healthy gut microbiome. Rather than try knocking them out all at once, feel free to incorporate one or two of these factors each week. For example, for the first week you can make a greater effort to avoid common food allergens, consume more fiber in week #2, etc.

If you can make these changes all at once then that's great, but even incorporating one or two of these tips each week can do wonders for your digestive health over time. So hopefully you realize how important it is not only to eat healthy, but to actually digest what you eat. I realize this might sound like common sense to you, but obviously it isn't something many people think about, or else acid-stopping drugs wouldn't be so popular.

Chapter Summary

- Eating whole foods and taking quality nutritional supplements won't do you much good if you aren't properly digesting what you consume.
- Millions of people take acid-stopping medication, which can interfere with their ability to digest the food they eat.
- Just beginning to eat well and taking quality supplements alone after years of eating junk food usually won't be enough to fix a digestive problem. However, it still is a good place to start.
- Make sure you read the seven tips I listed in this chapter to help improve your digestive health.

For access to the book references and resources, visit savemythyroid.com/hyperbooknotes

CHAPTER 10

The Immune-Gut Connection And Graves' Disease

DURING OUR FIRST consultation, Lana told me that she had cleaned up her diet, as she was eating only whole foods, and had completely cut out the refined foods and sugars. She had been gluten free for over one year, and was also dairy free. Other than some mild bloating every now and then she didn't experience any digestive symptoms, and she moved her bowels daily. In fact, after being diagnosed with hyperthyroidism she had more frequent bowel movements.

Upon doing an adrenal saliva test we found out that Lana had a very depressed Secretory IgA, which in many cases correlates with having a leaky gut, although it doesn't confirm this. I gave her some recommendations to help heal her gut, but she wanted to do further testing to confirm she had a leaky gut. And so I ordered the Intestinal Antigenic Permeability Screen from Cyrex Labs (their Array #2), which did confirm that she had a leaky gut.

I should mention that as of writing the third edition of this book I don't commonly recommend leaky gut testing, as these days I just assume that most people have a leaky gut. Anyway, Lana then followed my recommendations to heal her gut, and then she chose to retest the Array #2 from Cyrex Labs, which confirmed that her leaky gut had been healed. While healing her gut she also focused on correcting a few other imbalances she had, and eventually her thyroid panel and antibodies normalized.

As I discussed in Chapter 9, many people with hyperthyroidism have problems with digestion. In previous chapters I've already mentioned the term "leaky gut". This a condition that involves a compromised intestinal barrier, and as a result other proteins and larger molecules can pass through into the bloodstream.

Under normal circumstances, the spaces between the cells which line the small intestine are tight, and only certain substances can pass through. For example, potassium, sodium, and other minerals will pass through the intestinal lining through diffusion, while vitamins, minerals, amino acids, and other substances use active transport to pass through the intestinal cells.

What many people don't understand is that the health of the immune system is dependent on the health of the gastrointestinal tract. In the case of a leaky gut, when proteins and other molecules, as well as bacteria, pass through the small intestine into the bloodstream, this causes an immune system response. The reason for this is because these substances aren't supposed to be in the blood, and so the immune system treats them as being foreign, and therefore releases antibodies.

This in turn leads to inflammation, and this entire process can play a role in the development of autoimmunity and lead to a condition such as Graves' disease. So for anyone with Graves' disease, or any other autoimmune condition for that matter, restoring the health of the gut is essential.

How Does Someone Develop a Leaky Gut?

There are numerous factors which can lead to an increase in intestinal permeability (a leaky gut). Stress is one of the biggest factors, and these days most people deal with chronic stress on a daily basis. Stress of course can affect many of the systems in the body. This is why I constantly talk about the importance of improving your stress handling skills.

Poor diet is another potential cause of a leaky gut. People who eat a diet consisting of a lot of refined foods and sugars, as well as common allergens such as gluten, are more likely to develop this problem. Plus keep in mind that a poor diet will lead to nutritional deficiencies, which in turn can cause problems with the gut. For example, zinc, vitamin A, and vitamin B6 are very important for a healthy digestive system. As I already mentioned, food allergens can also cause a leaky gut. This is a big reason why people should consider avoiding gluten during the healing process, and is why some people might need to avoid other common food allergens, such as dairy.

Another factor that can lead to a leaky gut is a gut infection, such as H. pylori, or parasites. Small intestinal bacterial overgrowth (SIBO) or a Candida overgrowth can also cause a leaky gut. Heck, even mycotoxins from mold can potentially increase the permeability of the gut.[32]

Certain medications can also cause an increase in intestinal permeability. Examples of medications that can cause a leaky gut include antibiotics, proton pump inhibitors, NSAIDS, and even antithyroid medication. I actually spoke about the impact of methimazole and propylthiouracil (PTU) on the gut microbiome on my podcast, and if you want to learn more about this connection, including the research involved you can access this episode by visiting savemythyroid.com/25.

This doesn't mean that you shouldn't take any of these medications, as everything comes down to risks vs. benefits. This includes antithyroid medication, as while I personally used natural agents to manage my symptoms when I dealt with hyperthyroidism, there is a time and place for antithyroid medication.

What Are The Symptoms of a Leaky Gut?

First of all, it's important to understand that not everyone who has a leaky gut experiences digestive symptoms. With that being said, some potential symptoms include bloating, gas abdominal pain, bowel irregularities, joint pain, skin rashes, fatigue, and brain fog. Other symptoms can also be present due to this condition. But once again, it's important to understand that not everyone with a leaky gut has overt digestive symptoms. In the past when I did leaky gut testing I had numerous patients test positive for a leaky gut despite not having any digestive symptoms.

One of the symptoms I mentioned that could be associated with a leaky gut is brain fog, but there can be other causes of this, and one potential cause is a disrupted blood brain barrier. And the reason why I'm bringing this up here is that it's very common for people who have a disrupted intestinal barrier to also have a disrupted blood brain barrier.[33] I can't say that I commonly do testing for a "leaky brain", but Cyrex Labs does have a Blood Brain Barrier Permeability test.

Leaky Gut Testing Options

How can you determine if you have a leaky gut? If you have any type of digestive symptoms then this might be a sign that you have a leaky gut. Earlier I listed some of the symptoms that may be present when someone has a leaky gut. Another sign that someone has a leaky gut is if they have multiple food sensitivities.

Getting back to symptoms, as I mentioned earlier, symptoms alone won't reveal whether or not someone has a leaky gut. Testing is an option to consider, although there are limitations of the different tests. One of the markers I look for to help determine the state of someone's gut health is secretory IgA (SIgA), which is commonly depressed, although there are also situations when it is elevated. As I mentioned earlier, SIgA can be tested through either the saliva or the stool.

Testing for mannitol and lactulose can also help determine the presence of a leaky gut. This is done through the urine, as the person will drink a solution containing both of these water soluble molecules, and if high levels of lactulose is present, then this indicates an increase in intestinal permeability. Genova Diagnostics is one company that offers this test, although there are other companies that offer this type of testing as well. Just keep in mind that while an elevated lactulose confirms a leaky gut, false negatives are possible with this test.

I mentioned earlier that the company Cyrex Labs (www.cyrexlabs.com) has a test called the Intestinal Antigenic Permeability Screen. This is a blood test which looks at the different antibodies associated with an increase in intestinal permeability. When I used to recommend leaky gut testing I preferred using this test to determine whether someone had a leaky gut because it not only can tell if someone has a leaky gut by looking at Actomyosin and Occludin/Zonulin antibodies, but it can also determine the health of the gut flora by looking at the lipopolysaccharides (LPS). Lipopolysaccharides are also referred to as endotoxins, and they are large molecules found in gram-negative bacteria.

Zonulin is another biomarker of increased intestinal permeability. Elevated levels indicate the presence of a leaky gut. But once again, false negatives are common. While some comprehensive stool tests offer zonulin as an "add-on", I usually don't recommend testing it because if it's negative it doesn't rule out a leaky gut.

How Can a Leaky Gut Be Corrected?

A leaky gut can be challenging to heal, and there are a few reasons for this. First of all, it takes time for a leaky gut to develop, and as a result it will usually take at a few months to restore the health of the gut in most people. But a big reason why it can be challenging to heal the gut is because you first need to find the factors that caused the leaky gut.

This is yet another limitation of leaky gut testing, as none of the tests will determine the source of the leaky gut. Sometime it's as simple as eliminating common allergens from one's diet, including gluten and dairy. But if the cause is an underlying gut infection or environmental toxin then it can be more challenging to heal the gut.

What's The Deal With Food Sensitivity Testing?

Since certain foods can cause or contribute to a leaky gut and result in gut inflammation, you might wonder if food sensitivity testing is an option to consider. In fact, many natural healthcare practitioners will recommend for all of their patients to get tested for food sensitivities to determine which foods they can safely eat, and which foods they should avoid. When I was in chiropractic school I saw one of the teachers and did my very first food sensitivity test, and at the time I was fascinated how a simple test can tell me which foods my body was reacting too, and therefore should avoid. And let's face it, most of us would probably rather do such a test than go through an elimination diet, which I'll discuss in Chapter 11.

The problem is that most food sensitivity testing isn't completely accurate. This is especially true with IgG food sensitivity testing. False negatives are common with these tests, and so there is the chance they might continue eating a certain food which they tested negative for, even though they are sensitive to it. Sometimes a person will experience symptoms when eating something they're sensitive to, but other times they won't have any overt symptoms.

There is also a concern with false positives that may be caused by a leaky gut. So for example, if someone has a leaky gut and they choose to do an IgG food sensitivity test, they might notice that they test positive for dozens of foods, many of which are considered to be healthy. But if they were to do the same test a few weeks later it is very possible that they might test positive for foods that were previously negative, and vice versa.

That being said, there are times when I'll do IgG food sensitivity testing, but it usually is when someone is hitting a roadblock and I'm suspecting that there might be a healthy food they're eating and reacting to. And when recommending such a test I'll stick with certain labs, as not all labs that offer food sensitivity testing are created equally.

For example, one of the IgG food sensitivity panels I've recommended to my patients is the Multiple Food Immune Reactivity Screen from Cyrex Labs, which is also their Array #10. There are a few things I like about this test. One is that it tests both raw and cooked forms of common foods, as heating foods change its protein structure, and therefore changes its antigenicity. It also tests for the sensitivity to large gum molecules (i.e. xanthan gum).

I'll add that in 2022 I started using mediator release testing (MRT) on some of my patients. MRT is another type of food sensitivity test that determines how you react to different foods and food-chemicals. Unlike IgG food sensitivity testing, which measures antibodies, the MRT measures the release of mediators, which are inflammatory chemicals. An example of a mediator is histamine, although there are many more.

In addition to eating well and avoiding common food allergens, I just want to remind you that other factors might be affecting the health of the gut.

For example, if one's leaky gut is due to H. Pylori, parasites, or SIBO, just eating well and avoiding food allergens alone probably won't heal the gut. In the case of H. pylori, conventional medical treatment consists of the person taking two antibiotics (along with an acid-blocker), but this will compromise the gut even further. As I mentioned in Chapter 9, I try to take a more gentle approach when dealing with gut infections, as well as yeast and bacterial overgrowth.

Foods That Can Promote Gut Healing

While it's important to remove any factors that are causing the leaky gut, there are foods that can assist with gut healing. Bone broth is definitely one of the main ones, although I'll admit that when I dealt with Graves' disease I didn't drink bone broth. And the reason for this is that when I was dealing with Graves' disease back in 2008/2009, you didn't hear as much about bone broth as you do today.

And so I simply didn't know that bone broth would be beneficial, and therefore didn't drink it. These days not only do you see numerous brands of pre-packaged bone broth at local grocery stores, but even bone broth powders. Of course if you drink bone broth you want to make sure it's of good quality (i.e. organic chicken, 100% grass-fed cows).

Eating fermented foods can be beneficial to the gut microbiome and also help with gut healing. Examples of fermented foods you can eat include sauerkraut, fermented pickles, kefir, and kombucha. If you choose to drink kefir you might want to drink a non-dairy version of it, such as water or coconut kefir. Cabbage juice can also support gut healing.

Supplements and Herbs For Gut Healing

There are numerous supplements and herbs which can assist with gut healing:

1. **Prebiotics.** These provide food for the probiotic bacteria, and while I absolutely love probiotic supplements and have been taking them for years, over the last few years I've supplemented with prebiotics as well, specifically inulin and acacia fiber. If you experience digestive symptoms when consuming prebiotics it may be an indication of small intestinal bacterial overgrowth (SIBO).

2. **Probiotics.** These help to maintain a healthy gut environment. While I definitely encourage my patients to eat fermented foods, I also recommend probiotic supplements, and as I already mentioned, I personally take them as well. You just want to make sure you take one with well-researched strains, as there still are a lot out there that just list the species on the label. For example, Lactobacillus acidophilus is an example of a species, whereas Lactobacillus acidophilus LA-5 and LA-14 are considered to be specific strains. One of the probiotic supplements I recommend is called SMT-Probio, and I talk more about probiotic supplements in Chapter 12.

3. **Digestive enzymes.** Although not everyone needs to take digestive enzymes, I do find them helpful for many people. It's important to sufficiently break down the food you eat to prevent food sensitivities from developing. The digestive enzyme I recommend (Enzymes Plus) not only has digestive enzymes, but it also includes betaine HCL and ox bile.

4. **L-glutamine.** L-glutamine is an amino acid that is an energy source for cells in your small intestine. This provides nutrients to the gut to help the cells heal. You can take this alone, or as part of a gut healing formula.

5. **Other gut healing agents.** Some of the more common ingredients in gut healing formulas include deglycyrrhizinated licorice (DGL), aloe vera, zinc carnosine, N-Acetyl D-Glucosamine, marshmallow root, and slippery elm.

Will Healing The Gut Alone Cure Graves' Disease?

In my experience, restoring the health of the gut microbiome is a key factor when trying to regain your health. However, this doesn't mean that healing the gut alone will reverse Graves' disease. For example, if someone has compromised adrenals, then this probably needs to be addressed in order to achieve optimal health. Similarly, if someone has a toxic mold issue then this needs to be resolved

That being said, since an increase in intestinal permeability is part of the triad of autoimmunity, there is no question that in order to achieve a state of optimal health you need to heal the gut. And this isn't just the case with Graves' disease, but other hyperthyroid conditions as well. This is why I dedicated two chapters to the gut in this book, and easily could have included more.

In summary, the health of the immune system is dependent on the health of the gastrointestinal tract. Because of this, if someone has Graves' disease, restoring the health of the gut is essential. Just keep in mind that in order to heal the gut you need to find the factors that caused the leaky gut.

Chapter Summary

- Many people with hyperthyroidism and Graves' Disease have an unhealthy gut microbiome
- Since most of the immune cells are located in the gut, the health of the immune system is dependent on the health of the gastro-intestinal tract
- Some of the causes of a leaky gut include stress, poor diet, gut infections, and certain medications, including methimazole and PTU.
- Two specific tests for intestinal permeability are 1) the lactulose/mannitol test, and the 2) Intestinal Antigenic Permeability Screen by Cyrex Labs
- Some supplements and herbs which can assist with gut healing include probiotics, prebiotics, L-glutamine, DGL licorice, aloe vera, zinc carnosine, marshamallow root, and slippery elm.

For access to the book references and resources, visit savemythyroid.com/hyperbooknotes

CHAPTER 11

Hyperthyroid Diet Tips

Note: As of releasing the third edition of this book I'm also working on my next book, the title of which will be the "Hyperthyroid Healing Diet". My goal is to release this in the first quarter of 2024. And so while this chapter goes over the basics of a hyperthyroid healing diet, if you want greater detail and if you're reading this in early 2024 or beyond then you might want to check out my new book by visiting hyperthyroidhealingdietbook.com.

UPON REVIEWING THE CASE history of "Rachel", I noticed that she had numerous symptoms which indicated less than optimal digestive health. She experienced frequent bloating and gas, had indigestion on a regular basis, and while many people with hyperthyroidism experience more frequent bowel movements, Rachel was dealing with constipation. As a result, one of the primary areas I needed to help her support was her digestive health.

A big part of this involved dramatic changes in her eating habits, as she ate a horrible diet. While some people make abrupt changes to their diet, from our conversation I realized that Rachel wasn't ready to do this, and so I told her that I she can gradually begin incorporating more whole foods into her diet, and to greatly minimize the refined foods and sugars.

After a few weeks Rachel was eating much better. However, after a few months she wasn't receiving the results we both had hoped for. After some probing she finally admitted that she still started straying from the diet again. While there were other triggers and underlying imbalances we needed to address, I told her that eating well was an important piece of the puzzle.

So she set a goal for two weeks where at that time she would be eating only whole foods. It wasn't easy, but she was able to change her diet, and it wasn't too long before she began experiencing an improvement in her digestive symptoms (along with many of her other symptoms), followed by some positive changes in her thyroid blood tests and antibody levels. But I'm pretty sure she wouldn't have reached this point if she continued eating inflammatory foods on a daily basis.

When I was diagnosed with Graves' disease, proper nutrition definitely played a huge role in restoring my health. I probably don't need to inform you that different doctors will have varying opinions as to what is considered to be "healthy" with regards to one's diet. And let's be honest for a moment...nobody eats a "perfect" diet. In my opinion it's okay to indulge every now and then...after someone restores their health.

For example, I once consulted with a patient who loved milkshakes, which obviously isn't considered to be too healthy. This patient had about four or five milkshakes each week. And while I recommended for this person to completely eliminate milkshakes from his diet, I didn't tell him that he could never drink another milkshake after restoring their health. Of course I would hope that he would have a "healthier" milkshake in the future, and perhaps even use organic coconut milk in the future. And the same concept applies with other foods, as indulging every now and then after restoring one's health usually isn't a big deal.

Of course there are exceptions. For example, someone with Celiac disease probably won't be able to eat a gluten-based food "every now and then". And there are people who shouldn't have a milkshake every now and then, or an occasional slice of pizza, etc. And once again, during the hyperthyroid healing process it is important to be somewhat strict with the diet.

And so if you end up working with a natural healthcare practitioner, don't be surprised if he or she recommends for you to cut out all junk food during the healing process. This will probably include refined foods and sugars, fast food, unhealthy oils, etc. Some healthcare professionals will recommend for all of their patients to continue avoiding these foods after restoring their health.

Don't get me wrong, as it's not like I encourage people to eat unhealthy foods after they restore their health. And I don't want you to get the impression that I eat junk food on a regular basis, as overall I eat pretty healthy, but I can't say that since regaining my health I never eat any refined foods and sugars, never get exposed to gluten or dairy, etc. Once again, some people do need to strictly avoid certain food allergens on a permanent basis, but for many people, eating these foods on an occasional basis after they have restored their health usually won't cause them to relapse.

Important Rules To Any Hyperthyroid Healing Diet

In order to get the most out of any hyperthyroid healing diet, there are five important rules to follow:

Rule #1: The first rule is to minimize, or ideally completely eliminate refined foods and sugars while you are healing. One reason for this is because refined foods cause a spike in the blood sugar levels. As a result, if you eat refined foods frequently over a period of months and years, this will put a great deal of stress on your adrenals, as well as the pancreas. You want to focus on eating whole, healthy foods during the healing process.

Rule #2: Avoid common food allergens, including gluten, dairy, corn, and soy. I already discussed this in Chapter 9, as gluten is highly inflammatory, and the other three are problematic in a lot of people as well. One thing I didn't mention is how long you should avoid these food allergens.

Different practitioners will have different opinions. For example, many natural healthcare practitioners will advise their patients to avoid gluten on a permanent basis. This is especially true for those who have an autoimmune condition, which of course would include Graves' disease. In fact, some practitioners will recommend for all of their autoimmune patients to permanently avoid gluten, dairy, and grains (including corn).

There is a good argument for avoiding gluten permanently, although I can't say that I've been 100% gluten free since I've been in remission. I do try to avoid gluten most of the time, but occasionally I will have an exposure, and thankfully all has gone well, although that isn't the case with everyone. I also have dairy and grains occasionally, and find that many people are able to eventually reintroduce these.

I would recommend avoiding these common food allergens for at least 90 days. But there is a good argument that they should be avoided throughout the healing process. This is especially true with gluten, and many people also choose to avoid dairy, corn, and soy until they have restored their health. On the other hand, some people choose to reintroduce these before they have restored their health.

Rule #3: Avoid nightshades, grains, and legumes. I also discussed this in Chapter 9, and I mentioned how these aren't permanent eliminations. I recommend avoiding these for at least 30 days, although 90 days would be ideal. At this point you might be able to reintroduce them, although if you do this you will want to do so one at a time.

Rule #4: The fourth rule involves eating sufficient protein, and while this is important for everyone, since hyperthyroidism involves a loss of muscle mass, it's important that you eat enough protein on a daily basis. I recommend eating between 50% and 75% of your weight in protein per day. So for example, if you weigh 120lbs you would eat between 60 to 90 grams of protein per day.

Rule #5: The fifth and final rule is that you should eat a wide variety of plant-based foods. Keep in mind that I'm not recommending a vegan or vegetarian diet. But I would aim for at least 10 to 15 different fruits and vegetables each week, although more than this would be even better. And it's fine to gradually work up to this, as for example, if you're currently only eating five different vegetables per week then introduce one or two new ones every week until you reach 10 to 15.

Dealing With Insulin Resistance and Other Blood Sugar Imbalances

Insulin resistance occurs when the body becomes resistant to the effects of insulin. This is almost always caused by diet, and if unaddressed it can eventually lead to type II diabetes. Some people with thyroid and autoimmune thyroid conditions have insulin resistance, and the good news is that this condition can be reversed. In fact, most of the time type II diabetes can also be reversed through diet and lifestyle.

Before talking more about insulin resistance, it's probably a good idea to briefly discuss the role of insulin. Insulin is produced in the pancreas, specifically within the beta cells of the islets of Langerhans. Many people know that insulin is given to many diabetics to help lower their blood sugar levels. So without question, insulin plays a very important role in helping to balance the blood sugar levels. But in addition to this, it also has other functions. For example, insulin plays a role in DNA replication and protein synthesis. It also plays a role in lipid synthesis, along with the uptake of amino acids.

How does insulin resistance develop? As I briefly mentioned earlier, eating a poor diet is the main cause. And many of those who are trying to eat healthy are still consuming too many carbohydrates on a daily basis. For example, we all know that cookies, cakes, potato chips, candy, and many other foods are not good for us. Eating these foods on a regular basis is a big factor in the rise of insulin resistance and type II diabetes.

However, some people who avoid these foods still have problems with insulin resistance. I've consulted with people who are gluten free, yet are eating well over 300 grams of carbohydrates per day in the form of gluten-free grains (rice, oats, etc.), quinoa, potatoes, gluten-free pastas and bread, etc. So just because someone is avoiding pastries, potato chips, candy, pizza, and other junk food doesn't mean they are doing fine with their daily intake of carbohydrates.

How does insulin relate to thyroid health? Well, a few studies have linked hyperthyroid and hypothyroid conditions to insulin resistance.[34, 35] Yet another study links subclinical hyperthyroidism to insulin resistance.[36] The increased glucose associated with insulin resistance can cause a lot of problems. First of all, increased glucose can activate something called NF-kappaB, which can lead to inflammation. Second, insulin resistance also will activate adipocytes, making it difficult for people to lose weight. Finally, insulin resistance will upregulate the enzyme aromatase,[37] which can lead to estrogen dominance. While eating well is important to correct this condition, doing this might not correct the inflammatory process and/or estrogen dominance condition.

Weight loss is a classic symptom of hyperthyroidism, and if you've lost a lot of weight then you're probably not dealing with insulin resistance. However, it's not uncommon for people with hyperthyroidism to gain weight, even when not taking antithyroid medication. If this is the case then I would highly recommend testing the fasting insulin and hemoglobin A1C. Ideally you want the fasting insulin to be less than 5 µIU/mL and the hemoglobin A1C to be less than 5.2%.

Should You Test For Food Sensitivities?

I already discussed this in Chapter 10, as while I can't say that I never do food sensitivity testing, there are definitely limitations to this type of testing. This is especially true with IgG food sensitivity testing. I mentioned how in 2022 I started doing mediator release testing (MRT) on some patients, and so if someone absolutely wants to do a food sensitivity test this is currently what I'll recommend. Or if someone isn't progressing after a few months of care then this is also something to consider doing.

But for years I have recommended for people to start off with an elimination diet, and I still have my patients take this approach. It's not a perfect method of detecting food sensitivities, but the truth is that there is no perfect method out there.

Pros and Cons of an Elimination Diet

A less costly, and perhaps a more accurate approach than food sensitivity testing is an elimination diet, where you eliminate all of the common food allergens, along with other potentially problematic foods, and then slowly reintroduce them one at a time. There are different variations to doing this, but for my people with Graves' disease I commonly recommend an autoimmune Paleo (AIP) diet, which essentially serves as an elimination diet.

Here are the foods allowed on an AIP diet:

- Lean meats and poultry
- Organ meats
- Fish and many other types of seafood
- Fresh fruits
- Vegetables (excluding the nightshades)
- Healthy oils
- Spices
- Honey

So you would want to eliminate all other foods, and then slowly reintroduce foods one at a time, every three days. Dr. Sarah Ballantyne recommends to start by reintroducing foods that are more nutrient dense (i.e. egg yolks), and not reintroduce more problematic foods (i.e. nightshades) until later on.

AIP vs. Paleo Diet

While the AIP diet is a good starting point for those people with Graves' disease, we need to keep in mind a few things. First of all, it's a very restrictive diet, and some people won't be emotionally able to handle such a diet. Second, not all cases of hyperthyroidism are autoimmune in nature. So another option is to follow a standard Paleo diet, which is still a very healthy diet, and includes the following:

- Lean meats and poultry
- Organ meats
- Fish and many other types of seafood
- Eggs
- Fresh fruits
- Vegetables (excluding the nightshades)
- Nuts and seeds
- Healthy oils
- Spices
- Honey

So you can see that a standard Paleo diet is very similar to an AIP diet, with the main differences that it allows eggs, nuts, and seeds. So you'd still be avoiding grains, legumes, and dairy on this type of diet.

Can You Combine an Elimination Diet With Food Sensitivity Testing?

Earlier I mentioned how there is no perfect method for determining if someone has one or more food sensitivities. And so you might be wondering if you can do both an elimination diet and food sensitivity testing. This is an option to consider, although I can't say that I've done this with a lot of patients over the years, as I usually just start them out with an elimination diet, and then consider food sensitivity testing if they're not progressing as expected. And to be honest, even if they're not progressing as expected, a food sensitivity test isn't something I'll always recommend as a next step, as I very well might recommend a different type of test.

Anyway, if you choose to do an elimination diet and an IgG food sensitivity test, you would just want to make sure to do the blood draw before you start the elimination diet. And the reason for this is because IgG food sensitivity testing is measuring antibodies, and you need to be eating the food in order to have antibodies. For example, if you have a food sensitivity to tomatoes, and you cut out tomatoes from your diet, you no longer will be producing antibodies towards this food, and thus if you did the IgG food sensitivity test a few months later you would expect to have a negative result for tomatoes.

Just remember that tomatoes aren't avoided because of food sensitivities, but because of the compounds they and other nightshades have that can have a negative effect on gut health. And so if someone is eating tomatoes and tests negative on an IgG food sensitivity test (or a mediator release test), you would ideally still want to take a break from these. And the same concept applies to the other nightshades, as well as other foods that can be harsh on the gut.

On the other hand, with mediator release testing, it isn't necessary to be eating the food in order to get accurate results. And the reason for this is because unlike IgG testing, with mediator release testing you're not measuring antibodies. So for example, if you have an egg sensitivity and been avoiding eggs for a few months, we would expect an IgG test for eggs to be negative, whereas the MRT should pick up the food sensitivity.

What Foods Can a Vegetarian or Vegan Eat?

If you are a strict vegetarian or vegan, while you will avoid meat, poultry, and seafood, you of course still want to eat whole foods while avoiding the refined foods and sugars, unhealthy oils, etc. The concern with being a vegetarian, and especially a vegan, is that nutritional deficiencies are more likely to develop. One of the main reasons for this is because many vegans and vegetarians eat a lot of processed foods, although I'm sure there are many reading this who eat a healthy vegan or vegetarian diet. And if necessary you can supplement with certain nutrients.

I'll add that while I do think it's a good idea to avoid the grains while healing, some people do fine eating properly prepared legumes. One way to properly prepare them is through soaking, although another way is to pressure cook legumes. Doing this will help to reduce the lectins and other compounds that can interfere with gut healing.

Combining Diet with Detoxification

When I'm working with someone who has hyperthyroidism, after the first consultation I'll commonly recommend for them to make certain diet and lifestyle changes, and based on their health history, do certain tests to find their triggers and underlying imbalances. And at times I'll also recommend a program for them to support detoxification of their liver, lymphatics, kidneys, etc. So essentially they will be eating certain foods to support detoxification, mainly plenty of vegetables, and take certain supplements to help support detoxification.

Not surprisingly, I recommend that they purchase organic food, at least with regards to meat and produce. However, if they are on a strict budget, or if they live in an area where it's difficult to purchase organic foods, then they can visit the Environmental Working Group website (www.ewg.org)

and check out the Dirty Dozen and Clean Fifteen lists. The Dirty Dozen lists the top twelve fruits and vegetables with the greatest amount of pesticides, while the Clean Fifteen lists the top fifteen fruits and vegetables with the least amount of pesticides.

I'm sure there are some people reading this who will be overwhelmed just at the thought of going on an elimination diet, let alone combining an elimination diet with a detoxification. I will say that not everyone will do both, as the priority is definitely eating healthy. But if you're interested in the detoxification program I recommend you can visit savemythyroid. com/hyperbooknotes.

Put Together A Food Diary

Before beginning your "hyperthyroid healing diet", it's also a good idea to write down everything you eat for at least three days, and preferably one week. This not only includes the major meals you eat, but every snack, beverage, etc. This will make you more aware of what you're putting into your body, and if you're working with a natural healthcare professional then it will also provide them with valuable information as they assist you in the process of eating healthier. I ask all of my patients to do this before they consult with one of my certified health coaches about their diet.

After all, many of us think we're eating healthy, when in reality we're eating foods that aren't too good for us, are difficult to digest, etc. Years ago, one of my patients made me aware of a free program you can use by visiting www.myfitnesspal.com (there's also an application for smartphones). With this free program you can enter your food diary, and then it will give a breakdown of how many grams of proteins, fats, and carbohydrates you're consuming on a daily basis.

An Actual Example Of A Hyperthyroid Healing Diet You Can Follow

I know you're probably eager to know what a "healthy" diet is for someone who has hyperthyroidism. Keep in mind that someone who has Graves' disease might follow an AIP-type diet, while this might not be necessary for someone who has a non-autoimmune condition. I've decided to include an example of a daily hyperthyroid diet someone with Graves' disease would follow:

Breakfast: Smoothie which contains two cups of purified water, three to five cups of fresh vegetables (green and red leaf lettuce, arugula, collard greens, a stalk of celery) one half cup of mixed berries (raspberries, blueberries, and/or blackberries), a healthier protein powder, such as hydrolyzed beef, or a good quality pea protein (visit savemythyroid. com/hyperbooknotes for powders I use and recommend).

Mid-morning snack: small organic apple

Lunch: Grilled chicken salad: organic mixed greens, organic grilled chicken marinated in spices (i.e. parsley, oregano), olive oil and garlic as a dressing.

Mid-afternoon snack: another small smoothie

Dinner: Grass-fed burger (without the bun), one cup of steamed broccoli, one cup of roasted asparagus, a small sweet potato

This is a very simple version of the diet, and I realize that this will seem very restrictive for someone who is accustomed to eating a lot of refined foods and sugars, fast food, etc. And I do need to say that there is no diet that fits everyone perfectly, and if you have Graves' disease and this diet stresses you out then it's perfectly fine to eat more of a standard Paleo diet, which allows eggs, nuts, and seeds. I probably should mention that when I was dealing with Graves' disease in 2008/2009 there wasn't an AIP diet at the time, and so I followed a regular Paleo diet, minus the eggs (I wasn't much of an egg eater). And while I was progressing, eventually I hit a roadblock and ended up taking a two-month break from nuts and seeds.

I also should mention that it's not absolutely necessary to eat snacks in between meals. Intermittent fasting is definitely more popular now than when the first and second editions of this book came out, and so there might be people reading this who are tempted to get by with only two meals (i.e. lunch and dinner) and no snacks. You just need to be careful, as for many people with hyperthyroidism, intermittent fasting isn't a good fit.

This is especially true for those who have lost a lot of weight. For example, when I dealt with Graves' disease I lost 42lbs, and I definitely wouldn't have wanted to incorporate intermittent fasting back then. If you are gaining weight or are struggling to lose weight, then intermittent fasting might be something to consider, but you need to remember that it's important to get all of the macronutrients (especially protein) and micronutrients, which can be challenging with only two meals per day.

Once again, if you currently eat a lot of junk food and/or have strong sweet and carbohydrate cravings, I wouldn't expect you to change your eating habits overnight. Under such circumstances it is best to take it slow. I personally was brought up eating sugary cereals, plenty of fast food, and had soft drinks (punch, soda, etc.) on a daily basis. And while I was already eating much healthier when I was diagnosed with Graves' disease, it still wasn't an easy process. But knowing that this not only can help restore your thyroid health, but will also benefit your overall health, is a huge motivator.

Drink Plenty Of Purified Water

You also want to drink plenty of purified water, avoid any soft drinks, and even most juices, which can be high in sugar. As for what type of water you should drink, different natural healthcare practitioners have different opinions, but I recommend either water that has gone through a reverse osmosis process, or a good quality spring water (Mountain Valley Springs is an excellent quality spring water that comes in a glass bottle). Another good option is a whole house water filter, although you might need to purchase a separate fluoride filter.

With regards to the reverse osmosis water, some natural healthcare practitioners are concerned that it removes all of the minerals. Although you will get most of your minerals from the food you eat, if you're concerned you can add minerals to your water. Distilled water is another option to consider, and once again, if you're concerned about minerals being lost you can add minerals to your water. It's also worth mentioning that spring water such as Mountain Valley Springs is a good source of minerals.

It goes without saying that you should try everything you can to avoid tap water and water out of plastic bottles. Occasionally drinking from these sources isn't a big deal, but you definitely don't want to be drinking tap water daily, and the same goes for water out of plastic bottles. And if you are drinking water from a refrigerator filter in most cases it's similar to drinking tap water, other than the removal of chlorine.

Many people want to drink other beverages, and although I recommend to stick mainly with water, there are a few other options. Most herbal teas are fine to drink. As for green tea, I think this is fine, although for those with compromised adrenals I would recommend drinking an organic decaffeinated green tea. Drinking a cup or two of organic coconut milk per day is usually fine, although you do need to be careful about some of the ingredients, such as added gums. In the second edition of my book I mentioned the ingredient carrageenan, which at the time was included in many non-dairy beverages, including almond milk and coconut milk. Some studies show that carrageenan can lead to glucose intolerance and insulin resistance,[38] while other studies show that this ingredient can have harmful gastrointestinal effects.[39] The good news is that a lot of companies no longer use carrageenan.

As for coffee, I prefer for people to avoid drinking coffee at least initially while trying to heal, although I realize this isn't easy for some people to do, and it may take time for people to make this transition. In fact, some people find it more challenging to eliminate coffee than gluten and dairy.

Should People With Hyperthyroidism Consume Goitrogens?

Goitrogens interfere with the thyroid hormone production, which admittedly isn't as big of a factor in someone with hyperthyroidism as it would be with someone with a hypothyroid condition. In fact, one can make the argument that someone with hyperthyroidism should consume more goitrogenic foods in an attempt to lower their thyroid hormones. These are some of the foods that have goitrogenic properties:

- Soy (especially unfermented soy)
- Broccoli
- Brussels sprouts
- Cauliflower
- Kale
- Spinach
- Turnips
- Peaches
- Strawberries
- Pine nuts

The problem with intentionally using goitrogenic foods to lower thyroid hormones is that this approach doesn't work. And the reason I know this is because I tried doing this in practice, as when I first started working with pregnant women with hyperthyroidism, I realized that many didn't' want to take antithyroid medication, yet herbs such as bugleweed and motherwort aren't considered to be safe during pregnancy. And so I encouraged these women to eat a larger amount of raw goitrogenic vegetables to see if this would lower their thyroid hormones, but unfortunately this wasn't the case.

As a result, whether someone has hyperthyroidism or hypothyroidism, I encourage them to eat cruciferous vegetables on a regular basis. And if there is still concern on your part you of course can always cook them, as you don't need to eat them raw.

Looking For Recipes?

Both my wife and I are admittedly not very creative when it comes to creating new recipes. But if you're looking for specific recipes then I would recommend the following books:

- The Paleo Approach Cookbook by Dr. Sarah Ballantyne
- The Autoimmune Paleo Cookbook by Mickey Trescott
- Nourishing Traditions by Sally Fallon
- The Primal Blueprint Cookbook by Mark Sisson
- The Paleo Diet by Loren Cordain
- Gut and Psychology Syndrome by Natasha Campbell-McBride

Not all of these are cookbooks, but they all include numerous recipes. For example, while the first two books I listed have plenty of recipes, the book "Gut and Psychology Syndrome" only has one chapter dedicated to recipes. There are of course other good books besides the ones I listed, but these are the main ones I use.

Where Should You Shop?

As for where should you buy your food, although you can shop at your local health food store (we have one called Earth Fare), and I also do a lot of shopping at Whole Foods and Trader Joes, and there's also a Sprouts located about 30 minutes away. These days it's also common for conventional grocery stores to carry organic food, and even retail stores like Wal-Mart and Target. You might also want to check out Thrive Market (www.thrivemarket.com).

So hopefully you now have a better idea as to which foods you should eat for your hyperthyroid condition. Truth to be told, most people should eat a healthy diet consisting of whole foods, regardless of whether or not they have hyperthyroidism. Doing so can help prevent the development of such conditions, along with incorporating other lifestyle factors, such as exercising regularly, obtaining quality sleep, and doing a good job of managing stress. But for someone with hyperthyroidism or Graves" Disease, eating well can definitely help to improve their health, and is thus extremely important.

Chapter Summary

- Different doctors will have varying opinions as to what is considered to be "healthy" with regards to one's diet.
- Important rules to any hyperthyroid healing diet include 1) avoid refined foods and sugars, 2) avoid common food allergens, 3) avoid nightshades, grains, and legumes, 4) eat sufficient protein, and 5) eat a wide variety of plant-based foods.
- Many doctors test for food sensitivities, and while IgG food sensitivity testing or mediator release testing (MRT) are options to consider, for years I've had my patients follow an elimination diet.
- Before beginning your hyperthyroid healing diet, it's also a good idea to put together a food diary where you write down everything you eat for at least one week
- Even though goitrogens can potentially interfere with thyroid hormone production, in my experience, intentionally eating goitrogenic foods won't significantly lower thyroid hormone levels.

For access to the book references and resources, visit
savemythyroid.com/hyperbooknotes

CHAPTER 12

Nutritional Supplements & Herbs For Hyperthyroidism & Graves' Disease

CARLY WAS TAKING A FEW different nutritional supplements before I consulted with her. She was taking a multi-mineral vitamin, a calcium supplement, fish oils, and she was also taking a thyroid calming supplement that she had purchased online. The thyroid calming supplement consisted of some of herbs which typically help with hyperthyroidism (bugleweed, motherwort, lemon balm, etc.), along with some other ingredients. She had been on the thyroid calming supplement for about three months, and although initially taking this supplement helped with some of her hyperthyroid symptoms, she was looking to do more than just manage her symptoms naturally.

Based on her health history I recommended some testing, which included an adrenal saliva test, hair mineral analysis, comprehensive stool panel, and some blood tests. I then gave her specific recommendations based on the results. As for the supplements she was taking prior to working with me, some of them were purchased at local retail stores, and didn't seem to be of the best quality.

Even though I always recommend specific supplement brands and dosing, I'm fine with people taking different brands as long as they are of good quality, and ideally third-party verified. Carly decided to take the ones I recommended, and when combined with the diet and lifestyle changes, she made wonderful progress, and eventually reached the point where she was able to wean off of most of the supplements.

For those people with hyperthyroidism looking to take a natural treatment approach, there are numerous nutritional supplements and herbal remedies which can assist in restoring their health. As you probably know by now, just taking supplements and herbs alone isn't enough to accomplish this. When I was diagnosed with Graves' disease, nutritional supplements and herbs definitely were an important part of the recovery process.

On the other hand, there were other factors which were equally important in restoring my health. So if you have skipped the other chapters in this book and directly went to this one just so you can see which supplements and/or herbs you should take, then I definitely would advise you to start reading this book from the very beginning.

In fact, around the time of rewriting this chapter for the third edition of my book, I received a random email from someone who purchased both my Thyroid Calming Bundle and Thyroid Eye Disease Bundle, but after a couple of months she was still taking methimazole to manage her symptoms. And while she did make some diet and lifestyle changes, many times you need to go beyond diet and lifestyle in order to find and remove your triggers and underlying imbalances, which is what I told her. Without question improving one's diet and lifestyle is a key component to healing, but if someone isn't improving with diet and lifestyle alone (along with some nutritional supplements), then this is an obvious sign that something is missing, and in this situation it probably is a good idea to work with a competent natural healthcare practitioner.

Nutritional Supplements and Herbs I Commonly Recommend

The following represent some of the nutritional supplements and herbs I commonly recommend to those with hyperthyroidism. Keep in mind that I never recommend for anyone to take all of these, and while some of these I recommend to most of my patients, others are based on the testing that I do. Also, while some of these I still take on a wellness basis, many of these are "temporary" supplements that should be discontinued as someone's health improves. And just a reminder that even though I give some "suggested doses", different people will require different dosages.

With regards to the herbs, although I'm not an herbalist, I have received a certificate in practical herbal therapy from the Australian College of Phytotherapy. This program was put together by Kerry Bone, who is an herbalist with over 30 years of experience. He is also the author of a few books, including "Principles and Practice of Phytotherapy" and "The Essential Guide To Herbal Safety".

Note: The doses I list are approximate ranges, and of course anyone with hyperthyroidism should consult with a competent healthcare professional before taking any of the following supplements.

1. **Bugleweed (Lycopus virginicus, Lycopus europeaus).** Bugleweed is a great herb that can benefit many people with hyperthyroidism, and this was perhaps the main herb that helped manage my symptoms when I was dealing with Graves' disease. Just like many other people who have a

hyperthyroid condition, the increased pulse rate and heart palpitations can be scary, and bugleweed did help with these symptoms and allowed me to avoid taking antithyroid medication. While many people can have their hyperthyroid symptoms managed with bugleweed, I've noticed that approximately 25% of people who take this herb don't notice much of a difference. This is especially true for some people who have severely elevated thyroid hormones.

Think of bugleweed as an "antithyroid herb"[40], as it can help to decrease the T4 levels, and might also affect the conversion of T4 to T3. I usually recommend a 1:2 liquid extract to my patients, and according to Kerry Bone the recommended dose is 2 mL to 6 mL per day, although there I times when I will exceed this dosage, and I personally took 5 mL twice per day when I dealt with Graves' disease.

2. **Motherwort (Leonurus cardiaca).** This is another great herb which can help with the cardiac symptoms associated with hyperthyroidism, as it can improve heart function and blood circulation. [41] Even though the bugleweed did a great job of managing my symptoms, as my heart rate and palpitations decreased dramatically upon taking it, I still was experiencing some palpitations after starting the bugleweed. But taking both bugleweed and motherwort together pretty much helped to eliminate the cardiac symptoms. Obviously everything else I was doing helped as well, but both bugleweed and motherwort played a big role in providing natural symptom management.

Think of motherwort as a "natural beta blocker". This isn't to suggest that it's as powerful as a beta blocker, but motherwort frequently does a good job of managing the cardiac symptoms. I recommend a 1:2 liquid extract to my patients, and according to Kerry Bone the recommended dose is 2 mL to 4 mL per day, although there are times when I will exceed this dosage.

3. **Lemon Balm (Melissa officinalis).** This is another common herb which is used to manage the symptoms of hyperthyroidism for a few different reasons. First of all, lemon balm inhibits TSH receptor binding, which causes decreased production of T3 and T4 in the thyroid gland.[42] In addition, lemon balm has a calming effect, and may offer support for those suffering with anxiety and/or insomnia.[43] Some people combine bugleweed, motherwort, and lemon balm in order to help manage their hyperthyroid symptoms.

4. **L-Carnitine.** This is another natural agent that can help with the hyperthyroid symptoms by inhibiting both T3 and T4 entry into the cell nuclei[44] In order for it to be effective higher doses are necessary, and according to the research, someone with hyperthyroidism may need to take 2 to 4 grams on a daily basis.[44] One study showed that L-carnitine might even be useful in some cases of thyroid storm[45], although since thyroid storm is considered to be a medical emergency I do think it would be wise to go see a doctor right away.

Some people have asked me whether it's okay to take acetyl-l-carnitine. Most of the studies show that L-carnitine tartrate helps with hyperthyroidism, but there is no harm in taking a supplement that also has acetyl-l-carnitine. I just wouldn't take a supplement that only has acetyl-l-carnitine if you're using it for hyperthyroid symptom management.

While L-carnitine can be taken with bugleweed, motherwort, and/or lemon balm, it can also provide benefits on its own. I personally didn't take L-carnitine when I was dealing with Graves', but the reason for this is because at the time I wasn't aware of the benefits it provided for those with hyperthyroidism. That being said, L-carnitine is part of my thyroid calming bundle, which you can check out by visiting thyroidcalmingbundle.com.

Can You Combine Natural and Conventional Symptom Management Agents?

Before I discuss some of the other supplements I commonly recommend, I did want to mention that I have had patients with hyperthyroidism take some of the natural agents I just mentioned, along with antithyroid medication or beta blockers. For example, if someone is taking antithyroid medication and they're still experiencing heart palpitations, in most cases it's fine if they add motherwort. Or if they have a challenge with insomnia they can take lemon balm at night. Another scenario is if someone can't tolerate antithyroid drugs, and so they're taking a beta blocker, then in this situation it's usually fine to also take bugleweed or L-carnitine.

Can someone take bugleweed or L-carnitine at the same time as antithyroid medication? I have had patients do this, as while I can't tell anyone to stop taking their medication, when the goal is to wean off of the medication sooner than later (under the guidance of the prescribing doctor), I've had some people take bugleweed and/or L-carnitine 45 to 60 minutes away from the medication. Then once the thyroid hormones decrease and the TSH increases, the prescribing doctor should decrease the dosage of the antithyroid medication while you remain on the bugleweed or L-carnitine.

5. **Selenium.** This mineral is very important when it comes to immunity, and so if you have an autoimmune condition such as Graves' disease you should make sure you are not deficient in this mineral. Numerous studies have shown that taking selenium for 12 months was effective in reducing thyroid antibodies.[46] A couple of other studies also show that supplementing with selenium can benefit people with Graves' disease.[47, 48]

In some cases eating a few raw Brazil nuts each day will provide you with plenty of selenium. The problem is that you don't know how much selenium you're getting in a single Brazil nut, and as a result, if someone has a selenium deficiency I usually recommend supplementation in the form of selenomethionine. The dose will depend on the person, although it's not uncommon for healthcare professionals to recommend 200 mcg to 400 mcg of selenium per day to their patients. You just need to be cautious, as it is possible to overdose with selenium, which is yet another reason why it's always wise to work with a competent natural healthcare practitioner.

6. **Magnesium.** Many people are also deficient in magnesium, which has many different roles in the body, and as a result, a deficiency in magnesium can lead to many different health issues, including muscle spasms and insomnia. Taking supplements also can help, although eating a diet consisting of a wide variety of whole foods will greatly help, including plenty of green leafy vegetables. But just as is the case with selenium, if someone is deficient in magnesium I usually recommend a supplement, such as SMT-Mag, which is a highly absorbable form of magnesium. If someone is experiencing constipation then magnesium citrate may be a better option.

As for how much to take, the dose can be anywhere from 200mg to 600mg, and in some cases higher than this. One way to know if you're taking too much magnesium is that your stools will become loose. Of course loose stools can also be caused by hyperthyroidism as well, and so if you're already experiencing loose stools prior to supplementing with magnesium it might be challenging to know if you are taking too much, and as a result, you might want to start with a lower dosage.

7. **Omega 3 fatty acids.** A lot of people take omega three fatty acids in the form of fish oils, but you do want to make certain of a couple of things. First of all, you want to make sure you take a high quality fish oil, as many of the fish oils sold in retail stores are rancid, which you

can usually tell if they have a "fishy" odor upon cutting the supplement open. Second, don't consume too high of a dosage, as while you definitely want to avoid a deficiency, at the same time you don't want to have an excess in your system, as this can lead to other health issues.

That being said, I usually recommend between 1,000 to 2,000 mg of eicosapentaenoic acid (EPA) and 500 to 1,000 mg of docosahexaenoic acid (DHA). You might be wondering about vegetarian sources of omega-3 fatty acids, such as chia seeds and flax seeds. Alpha-linolenic acid is the parent fatty acid found in chia seeds and flaxseed, but the problem is that there can be restricted conversion to EPA and DHA.[49]

I personally like to take both, as I take a fish oil supplement daily, and I also add a tablespoon of flax seeds to my smoothies (I purchase them whole and grind them). Some people have asked me about krill oil, and while there are a lot more studies showing the anti-inflammatory benefits of consuming fish oil, the studies on krill oil show that it is just as effective, and possibly even more effective.[50] But the problem with both krill oil and cod liver oil is that you would have to take a lot more than recommended to get enough EPA and DHA.

If you've been relying on vegetarian sources of omega-3 fatty acids, they you might want to consider doing a fatty acid profile, or at the very least, an omega-3 index. You ideally want the omega-3 index to be at least 8%, and so if it's lower than this then you might need to switch to a different source. You can learn more about the fatty acid profile I recommend by visiting savemythyroid.com/hyperbooknotes.

8. **Vitamin D.** Most people are vitamin D deficient, and a big reason for this is because many people don't get enough sun exposure, which is the best source of vitamin D. And many people who do get adequate sun exposure always put on sun block, which also blocks the absorption of

vitamin D. However, some people who get a lot of sun exposure without using sun block also are deficient in vitamin D, as I've consulted with many such patients. There can be numerous reasons for this, including a higher latitude, a lot of air pollution, or even a genetic polymorphism of the vitamin D receptors.

As a result, many people need to supplement with vitamin D3, but before you do this it is a good idea to get tested to confirm that you are indeed deficient in vitamin D. A vitamin D deficiency can cause a lot of problems, including a compromised immune system, which can eventually lead to the development of an autoimmune thyroid condition, increase the likelihood of certain cancers, as well as cause many other conditions. The Vitamin D Council shows some of the different conditions that a vitamin D deficiency can lead to:

"Current research has implicated vitamin D deficiency as a major factor in the pathology of at least 17 varieties of cancer as well as heart disease, stroke, hypertension, autoimmune diseases, diabetes, depression, chronic pain, osteoarthritis, osteoporosis, muscle weakness, muscle wasting, birth defects, periodontal disease, and more."

A typical lab reference range of the 25 hydroxy vitamin D test is 30 to 80 ng/ml, but while a level of 30 ng/ml might be sufficient for bone health, it is less than optimal for immune system health. And this isn't just my opinion, as there are studies which reveal this, and you can learn a lot more by visiting the Vitamin D Council website, or reading some research articles on Pub Med. As for the dose I recommend to my patients, this does depend on how deficient someone is, as if someone has a severe deficiency I might have them take doses as high as 10,000 IU/day for a few months, while in other cases I'll have them supplement with 2,000 to 5,000 IU/day. I will then have them retest after three to six months.

Some people are concerned about taking higher doses of vitamin D3, but according to a study, intake of greater than 1,000 IU has been avoided even though the weight of evidence shows that the currently accepted, no observed effect limit of 2,000 IU/day is too low by at least 5-fold.[51] Another study confirmed this.[52] That being said, I recommend to consult with a healthcare professional before supplementing with higher doses of vitamin D3.

One more thing I need to mention is that if you supplement with vitamin D3, you should also take vitamin K2. And the reason for this is because while vitamin D increases the intestinal absorption of calcium, vitamin K2 helps to guide the calcium into the bone. If you're deficient in vitamin K2 then calcium might get deposited into some of the soft tissues of the body, including the arteries. The good news is that a lot of vitamin D3 supplements also have vitamin K2 added, but if necessary you can always take a separate vitamin K2 supplement.

9. **Probiotics.** Even though I have probiotics listed towards the end of this list, I consider it to be one of the more important supplements. I've been taking probiotic supplements for many years, and recommend one to just about everyone. And it's not just about gut health, as probiotics can also modulate the immune system.[53] In fact, some research suggests that they can increase regulatory T cells, which can help to suppress autoimmunity.[54]

What you need to know about probiotics is that many companies still only list the species on the bottle, but you want to make sure to take one with well-researched strains. As an example, "lactobacillus" is a genus, whereas "lactobacillus acidophilus", is a species. On the other hand, "lactobacillus acidophilus LA5" is a specific strain. And the reason why this is important is that different strains have different functions.

How important is the potency, or colony forming units (CFU)? Although I usually recommend a probiotic supplement with 30 to 50 billion CFU, the specific strains are more important. In other words, it would be more beneficial to take a 10 billion CFU probiotic supplement with well-researched strains than a 50 billion CFU probiotic supplement that just listed the species on the bottle. SMT-Probio is an example of a high-CFU probiotic with well-researched strains.

10. **Digestive enzymes.** I also commonly recommend digestive enzymes to my patients, but unlike probiotic supplements, I can't say that I take digestive enzymes daily on a wellness basis. But a lot of people have impaired digestion and low stomach acid, and so I usually will recommend a digestive enzyme supplement that not only has enzymes, but also a small amount of betaine HCL and some ox bile. If someone has healthy levels of HCL they usually will do fine on this, but if they have excessive HCL levels then of course there are digestive enzymes that don't include betaine HCL.

But how does someone know if they have low stomach acid levels, and therefore need to take something like betaine HCL? Unfortunately there is no perfect test out there. The Heidelberg Stomach Acid Test can help to determine if someone has hypochlorhydria, which is low stomach acid. This involves the patient swallowing a capsule which includes a pH monitoring device, and this measures the levels of stomach acid while the person drinks a baking soda solution. However, getting a doctor to order this test isn't always easy.

Some natural healthcare professionals will recommend a "betaine HCL challenge", which involves taking a capsule of betaine HCL with pepsin, along with a high protein meal, and if someone doesn't notice any symptoms (i.e. heartburn) then this is usually an indication that the person has low stomach acid. On the other hand, if the person experiences heartburn then this is a sign that they have sufficient levels of stomach acid. I should also mention that while I commonly recommend betaine HCL, digestive bitters can also be helpful to stimulate your own body's stomach acid production.

Other Supplements And Herbs To Consider

B vitamins. There are many different conditions in which deficiencies of the B vitamins can lead to, and so obviously you want to make sure you avoid such a deficiency. Trying to get as many of the B vitamins through diet is ideal, but if stress is a big factor in your life then you might benefit from taking a B complex. On the other hand, if you have a problem with methylation then you might benefit from taking methylated folate or vitamin B12 (methylcobalamin).

I'm not going to get into great detail when it comes to methylation in this book, but methylation is necessary when it comes to protein synthesis, detoxification, the formation of neurotransmitters, the regulation of hormones, and it has numerous other functions. One way to determine if you have a methylation problem is if you have elevated homocysteine levels, which you can test for through the blood. I had elevated homocysteine levels in the past, and through genetic testing I found out that I had a homozygous C677T genetic polymorphism, which is a common genetic variation. As a result, I take a methylation supplement on a wellness basis in order to keep my homocysteine at a healthy level.

CoQ10. Hyperthyroidism is associated with enhanced oxidative stress involving enzymatic and non-enzymatic antioxidants.[55] Hyperthyroidism is also linked with reduced circulating levels of CoQ10.[56] A study looked at the circulating levels of CoQ10 in both hypothyroid and hyperthyroid conditions, and found that the values of CoQ10 in hyperthyroid patients are among the LOWEST in different human diseases.[57]

In addition, another study shows that thyroid hormones have a profound effect on mitochondrial oxidative activity, and that hyperthyroid muscular tissues undergo several biochemical changes that predispose them to free radical-mediated injury.[58] Yet another study confirmed that serum CoQ10 levels in hyperthyroidism were significantly lower than that of euthyroid subjects, while in hypothyroidism, serum CoQ10 levels did not show any significant difference from that of euthyroid subjects.[59]

Truth to be told, when I was diagnosed with Graves' disease I wasn't aware of these studies involving CoQ10, and so I didn't take it. As a result I can't say that taking CoQ10 is essential for someone looking to restore their health. And one of my goals is to limit the number of nutritional supplements someone is taking, but based on the studies I discussed taking CoQ10 is something to consider if you have hyperthyroidism, which probably is the case if you're reading this book.

This especially is true for those people with hyperthyroid conditions who are on beta blockers. Numerous studies have shown that beta blockers such as Propranolol can inhibit mitochondrial CoQ10 enzymes.[60, 61] As a result, anyone who is taking beta blockers might want to consider taking CoQ10, regardless of whether or not they have hyperthyroidism.

In addition to beta blockers, it is well known that statins (cholesterol lowering medication) also interfere with the synthesis of CoQ10.[62] And so people taking statins might also want to consider taking CoQ10. In fact, one study showed that CoQ10 supplementation prevents both plasma and platelet CoQ10 decrease, without affecting the cholesterol lowering effect of the drug.[63] In most cases of hyperthyroidism I would recommend a minimum of 100mg of CoQ10 per day, and in some cases taking between 200mg and 400mg per day might be necessary.

Iron. It's also common for people with hyperthyroid conditions to have an iron deficiency. Many natural healthcare practitioners overlook this as a cause of the patient's fatigue. Although compromised adrenal glands can lead to fatigue, certain deficiencies can also cause this, such as iron. Keep in mind that not all anemia is due to iron, as there are other reasons why someone might have anemia. But I think it's a good idea for most people to get a full iron panel consisting of serum iron, ferritin, iron saturation, and total iron binding capacity.

A low ferritin is usually the first sign of an iron deficiency, but keep in mind that the inflammation associated with Graves' disease may raise the ferritin levels, which is why it's a good idea to also look at the TIBC and iron saturation. Plus, even if someone is low in iron, one wants to find out why this is the case, as while it might be due to low iron intake, there can be other factors, including heavy menstrual bleeding, hypochlorhydria (low stomach acid), a vitamin C deficiency, and absorption problems. Another reason to do an iron panel is that some people have elevated iron markers, which sometimes can be related to hyperthyroidism, but other times can be a genetic condition called hemochromatosis.

Gamma-Linolenic Acid (GLA). GLA can also help with the inflammation, and will produce different prostaglandins than omega-3 fatty acids. Some sources of GLA include borage oil, black currant seed oil, and evening primrose oil. I typically will recommend between 150mg to 300mg of GLA to my patients, and commonly have them take this every other day.

Copper. Some people with hyperthyroidism and Graves' disease have a copper deficiency, and these people of course should supplement with a small amount of copper (i.e. 1 or 2 mg/day). However, it also isn't uncommon for someone to have a copper toxicity problem, which is why someone shouldn't just be given copper randomly. As usual, proper testing is necessary to determine whether someone is deficient in copper, or has a copper toxicity problem. Copper has many different roles, as it's important for immunity, as well as the health of the thyroid and adrenal glands.

Lithium. Although I prefer bugleweed and L-carnitine as natural anti-thyroid agents, lithium can affect the production of thyroid hormone in multiple ways. First of all, lithium inhibits iodine uptake, and iodine is important for the formation of thyroid hormone. It also inhibits iodo-tyrosine coupling, alters thyroglobulin structure, and inhibits thyroid hormone secretion.[64] Lithium also decreases peripheral deiodination of thyroxine (T4) by decreasing the activity of type I 5' de-iodinase enzyme.[65] In other words, it affects the conversion of T4 to T3.

Most of the studies involving lithium's antithyroid properties used lithium carbonate. However, a medical doctor would need to prescribe lithium carbonate, and most will be unwilling to do this for managing the hyper-thyroid symptoms. Lithium orotate can be purchased over-the-counter, but it's unclear exactly how much someone with hyperthyroidism can safely take without putting significant stress on the kidneys.

An older study looked at kidney function and lithium concentrations of rats given lithium orotate or lithium carbonate, and found that lithium orotate had a negative effect on kidney function,[65] but besides this being an animal study, a more recent study showed that chronic use of lithium at low doses did not affect renal function and was clinically safe.[66] I did come across one lithium orotate toxicity case study involving an 18-year old woman, [66] although she took 18 tablets of lithium orotate, which definitely is not recommended!

Detox supplements. In some cases, taking supplements to reduce one's toxic load can be beneficial. More and more people are aware of the benefits of glutathione, which is a powerful antioxidant. Glutathione combines with vitamin E and selenium to form glutathione peroxidase, which helps to protect the thyroid gland from oxidation damage.

Glutathione plays important roles in antioxidant defense, nutrient metabolism, and regulation of cellular events (including gene expression, DNA and protein synthesis, cell proliferation and apoptosis, signal transduction, cytokine production and immune response, and protein glutathionylation).[69] The body produces glutathione on its own, but certain factors such as stress, poor diet, environmental toxins, and other factors deplete glutathione levels.

Although many people have low glutathione levels, and taking liposomal or acetylated glutathione can help raise these levels, another option is to take the precursors of glutathione. Eating cruciferous vegetables (broccoli, kale, cauliflower, etc.) can help to boost the glutathione levels. Consuming a healthy form of whey protein can also increase the glutathione levels, but the problem is that myself and many other practitioners advise their autoimmune patients to avoid dairy. With regards to supplements, selenium, N-acetyl-cysteine, and alpha lipoic acid can increase glutathione levels, as well as milk thistle. Mild to moderate exercise can also help to boost glutathione levels.

Schisandra and burdock can also help with detoxification. Schisandra (Schisandra chinensis) has been used for centuries as a plant of traditional Chinese medicine, and the lignans of schisandra has been investigated in hundreds of studies that have confirmed adaptogenic effects, central nervous system stimulation, hepatoprotective effects and potential anticancer potential (68). Burdock has been used therapeutically in Europe, North America and Asia for hundreds of years. In the root, the active ingredients have been found to "detoxify" blood and promote blood circulation, and antioxidants and antidiabetic compounds have also been found.[70] In the seeds, some of the compounds possess anti-inflammatory effects.[71] Another study showed that burdock root tea significantly decreased the levels of hs-CRP, which is an inflammatory marker.[72]

Turmeric/Curcumin. Turmeric has many different benefits, but one of the main benefits with regards to Graves' disease is to help support the inflammatory response. Numerous studies have shown how turmeric decreases the amount of pro-inflammatory cytokines, resulting in a decrease in inflammation.[73, 74, 75]

Resveratrol. Resveratrol also can help greatly with the inflammation, as demonstrated by several studies.[76, 77, 78] Resveratrol can also help to inhibit the aromatase enzyme, thus helping with conditions such as estrogen dominance.[79] And there is also evidence that it can reduce oxidative stress in those with thyroid eye disease.[80]

Herbs for adrenal support. There are many herbs that can support the hypothalamic-pituitary-adrenal (HPA) axis, including ashwagandha, eleuthero, holy basil, and rhodiola. I absolutely love ashwagandha, although it is somewhat controversial in those with hyperthyroidism. The same can be said with the herb eleuthero, also known as Siberian Ginseng, which is what I took when I dealt with Graves' disease. The concern with both ashwagandha and eleuthero is that they also support the hypothalamic-pituitary-thyroid (HPT) axis, and in some people can potentially increase thyroid hormone production, which isn't what you want in someone who has hyperthyroidism.

In addition, ashwagandha is a member of the nightshade family. And while supplementing with ashwagandha probably isn't as harsh on the gut as eating tomatoes, eggplant, and other nightshade foods, some people still don't do well with it. That being said, while you might want to be cautious about taking a separate ashwagandha supplement, one of the products I commonly recommend for those with high cortisol levels has some ashwagandha in it, and most people with hyperthyroidism do fine with it. But you can improve your adrenal health without taking ashwagandha.

There are other supplements and herbs which can benefit people with hyperthyroidism. For example, some people can benefit from taking a high potency multivitamin, and if you want to know what I commonly recommend you can visit savemythyroid.com/hyperbooknotes. The goal here isn't to list every single nutritional supplement and herb which can benefit people with hyperthyroid conditions, but I did try to list the most important ones.

How can you determine which of these supplements you need to take? While there are a few general supplements I commonly recommend to people with hyperthyroidism, I usually determine which supplements someone has to take through a combination of the person's health history and through testing for triggers and underlying imbalances. After all, a lot of people are already taking a lot of supplements prior to working with me, and while I have my favorites, my goal isn't to simply add to their list, as I want to make sure they're taking what they need in order to help restore their health.

I do want to remind you that while I recommend nutritional supplements and herbs, in all likelihood you'll need to do more than take supplements to restore your health. And the reason why I'm mentioning this here is because it's common for me to consult with someone who has been taking a dozen or more different supplements prior to seeing me, and while sometimes the supplements were recommended by a different healthcare practitioner, many times they're doing this on their own. Once again, I like supplements and recommend them, but taking more supplements isn't necessarily the answer to restoring your health.

This is yet another reason why it's wise to consult with a competent natural healthcare practitioner who has experience working with hyperthyroid patients, as they will evaluate your condition and give specific recommendations depending on which triggers and underlying imbalances you have. Not only that, but they will also monitor your progress so that you're not taking these supplements longer than you need to. As I mentioned earlier, some of these supplements can and should be taken regularly (fish oils, magnesium, etc.), but others do not need to be taken long-term. So rather than taking these supplements and herbs on your own, do yourself a favor and consult with a natural healthcare practitioner.

What About Iodine?

Since there is a great deal of controversy when it comes to iodine supplementation and thyroid health, I've decided to dedicate an entire chapter on iodine. I'll tell you here that over the years my stance on iodine supplementation has changed, as in the past I commonly recommended iodine testing and supplementation to most of my patients, but this definitely isn't my approach now. Although in some cases supplementing with high-dose iodine can lower thyroid hormones, it can also have the opposite effect, and can potentially exacerbate the autoimmune response in those people with Graves' disease. For more information on iodine refer to Chapter 13.

Be Cautious When Combining Antithyroid Herbs and Prescription Drugs

If you are currently taking antithyroid medication such as methimazole or PTU, you need to be careful about adding natural antithyroid agents such as bugleweed and L-carnitine. If you take too high of a dose of methimazole or PTU this can make you hypothyroid. Similarly, if you take bugleweed and/or higher doses of L-carnitine along with antithyroid medication it can also make you hypothyroid. Most of the time the hypothyroidism is reversible, but you still need to be careful, which is another reason to work with an expert when taking these supplements and herbs.

Chapter Summary

- For those people with hypethyroidism looking to take a natural treatment approach, there are numerous nutritional supplements and herbal remedies which can help assist in restoring their health back to normal.
- Although taking nutritional supplements and herbs can be beneficial, they're not a replacement for eating healthy, managing one's stress, etc.
- The following are some of the nutritional supplements and herbs I recommend for those with hyperthyroidism: 1) bugleweed, 2) motherwort, 3) lemon balm, 4) L-carnitine, 5) selenium, 6) magnesium, 7) fish oils, 8) vitamin D, 9) probiotics, and 10) digestive enzymes.

For access to the book references and resources, visit
savemythyroid.com/hyperbooknotes

CHAPTER 13

The Truth About Iodine And Hyperthyroidism

MANY PEOPLE WITH THYROID and autoimmune thyroid conditions are told to avoid iodine, and this includes those with hyperthyroidism. Not only are they usually advised not to take any iodine supplements, but many are told to avoid food sources of iodine. The main reason for this is because many doctors assume that people with an overactive thyroid have an excessive amount of iodine. And the reason for this is because iodine is essential for the production of thyroid hormone, and so if the thyroid gland is producing an excessive amount of thyroid hormone, as is the case with conditions such as Graves' disease and toxic multinodular goiter, then it's easy for someone to assume that there is also an excess amount of iodine.

Before I go any further, I need to let you know that my thoughts on iodine has without question changed since writing the 2013 edition of this book. Back then I was in favor of testing everyone for an iodine deficiency, and then having them supplement with iodine if they were deficient. The problem with this approach is that 1) there are limitations with the types of testing available, and 2) iodine can sometimes worsen a person's hyperthyroid condition, which I'll talk about more in this chapter.

Keep in mind that while I'm cautious about people with hyperthyroidism supplementing with iodine, this doesn't mean that I've switched from being "pro-iodine" to "anti-iodine". I don't advise people to avoid all food sources of iodine, and I'm usually not concerned about iodine in a multivitamin. But I do get concerned when someone takes a separate iodine supplement, and I'm also cautious about them eating very high food sources of iodine, such as sea vegetables.

My Personal Experience With Iodine Supplementation

When I took a natural treatment approach for my Graves' disease condition, the healthcare practitioner I was working with recommended for me to supplement with higher doses of iodine. Before doing this she recommended for me to do a 24-hour iodine loading test, which involves taking a 50 mg tablet which consists of iodine and potassium iodide prior to collecting the urine samples. After a deficiency was discovered I began supplementing with a product called Prolamine Iodine, as I started by taking a 3mg tablet each day (since then the tablets have been decreased to 600 mcg), and I gradually increased the dosage until I was taking three tablets three times per day, for a total of 27mg. I don't remember exactly how long I took this dosage of iodine for, but it was for at least a few months, and I eventually did a retest of the iodine loading test, and upon seeing an improvement I began weaning myself off of the iodine.

I did very well when taking the iodine, and I didn't experience any adverse effects. And when something works well for you, it's natural to assume that the same approach will work for others with similar conditions, and so when I initially began helping people with thyroid and autoimmune thyroid conditions I would recommend for just about all of my patients to do a urinary test for iodine, and if they were deficient I would have them supplement with iodine. However, I would also have them take certain precautions, which I'll discuss later in this chapter.

Of course supplementing with iodine wasn't the only thing I did when I took a natural treatment approach, as I ate whole healthy foods, did things to manage my stress, took supplements to support my adrenals and gut, etc. And so I don't think the iodine was the main factor responsible for my recovery. And the reason I'm confident in saying this is because for a number of years now I haven't routinely recommended iodine testing and supplementation to my patients, yet most people are successful in restoring their health.

My Patient's Experience With Iodine

Although I've seen many people with hyperthyroidism receive amazing results without supplementing with iodine, in the first few years of my practice I commonly recommended iodine testing and supplementation. And I will admit that most of my patients seemed to tolerate iodine quite well. That being said, not all of them did well with iodine supplementation. But my perspective of iodine really began to change when I started attending nutritional conferences taught by healthcare practitioners who presented research about the risks of iodine triggering an autoimmune thyroid condition. This was especially true with regards to Hashimoto's thyroiditis, but iodine supplementation can also be a concern with Graves' disease.

That being said, since I received good results with most of my thyroid and autoimmune thyroid patients, and since many of my patients supplemented with iodine at the time, not surprisingly I was resistant to stop recommending iodine testing and supplementation to my patients. However, it was hard to argue with the research, as some studies show a higher incidence of autoimmune thyroiditis in populations that were exposed to iodine.[81,82] However, there is also some evidence that the reason for this might be due to these populations being deficient in selenium.

The Connection Between Selenium and Thyroid Autoimmunity

But how can being deficient in selenium increase the risk of developing thyroid autoimmunity? Well, hydrogen peroxide plays a role in the oxidation of iodide to iodine. And it is well known that hydrogen peroxide is a source of free radicals.[83, 84] These free radicals cause an increase in proinflammatory cytokines, which is a factor in autoimmune conditions such as Graves' disease.

Selenium is important for the formation of selenoproteins. These selenoproteins are powerful antioxidants, and they help to neutralize the effects of oxidative stress by reducing these free radicals. So if someone has a selenium deficiency, this will result in a decrease in selenoproteins, and this in turn will cause an accumulation of hydrogen peroxide, which will produce more free radicals, and this results in a greater number of proinflammatory cytokines, etc.

As a result, anyone who supplements with iodine will also want to make sure they have healthy levels of selenium. Taking 200 mcg of selenium per day is commonly recommended. Other nutrients which can also be beneficial include vitamin C, magnesium, and the B vitamins.

What Are The Health Benefits of Iodine?

Although this chapter might seem to be negative towards iodine, the truth is that iodine has numerous health benefits. Here are some of the more important ones:

1. **Iodine is important for the production of thyroid hormone.** So while you don't want to have an excessive amount of iodine, an iodine deficiency also isn't a good thing.

2. **Iodine helps with the detoxification of halides.** Bromide, fluoride, and chloride have chemical structures similar to iodine, and thus they compete for the same receptor sites. As a result, being exposed to larger amounts of fluoride, bromide, or chloride can result in an iodine deficiency. On the other hand, supplementing with iodine can displace these other halides from the receptors, which is a good thing since these other halides have toxic effects.

3. **Iodine has antimicrobial properties.** Many people reading this know that iodine makes a great antiseptic. Iodine is bactericidal, fungicidal, tuberculocidal, virucidal, and sporicidal (10). The antimicrobial action of iodine is rapid, even at low concentrations, as iodine rapidly penetrates into microorganisms and attacks key groups of proteins, nucleotides, and fatty acids, which results in cell death.[85]

4. **Iodine plays a role in regulating estrogen metabolism.** Iodine modulates the estrogen pathway, which seems to explain why those who consume larger amounts of iodine have a reduced risk of developing breast and prostate cancer.[86, 87] And as I'll discuss in Chapter 21, problems with estrogen metabolism can also be a factor in the development of thyroid nodules, although I should add that an iodine deficiency isn't the only cause of having estrogen metabolism issues.

5. **Iodine can help prevent damage from radiation exposure.** Iodine supplementation can prevent the negative effects caused by radiation, as it helps to block radiation from being absorbed by the thyroid gland.

5 Reasons Why Some People Experience Problems With Iodine Supplementation

Once again, I'm very cautious these days when it comes to iodine supplementation. But I still wanted to explain some of the different reasons why someone might experience negative effects when supplementing with iodine. When someone with hyperthyroidism supplements with iodine and doesn't do well, there are typically five main reasons for this:

1. **They don't have an iodine deficiency.** Although some people are deficient in iodine, the truth is that not everyone has an iodine deficiency. This is why I recommend urinary testing before anyone supplements with iodine, although you need to keep in mind that there are limitations to such testing, and even if someone is truly deficient in iodine they might not do well for some of the other reasons I'm about to discuss.

2. **They are taking too large of a dose.** Some people supplement with very large doses of iodine. And while some people might do well on very high doses of iodine, everyone is different. For example, one person might feel great taking 25 to 50mg of iodine, while another person feels awful when taking a much lower dose. Of course one has to keep in mind that you can't always go by symptoms, and so just because someone feels great taking larger doses of iodine doesn't mean that it's not causing an increase in oxidative stress.

3. **They have low levels of antioxidants.** As I mentioned earlier, having low levels of selenoproteins can lead to an increase in oxidative stress and free radicals upon supplementing with iodine. Taking selenium with

iodine might help, but sometimes doing so isn't sufficient, and this is especially true when supplementing with very high amounts of iodine.

4. **They experience a "detox" reaction.** This actually can be a potential benefit of iodine supplementation, as it competes with some of the more harmful halides, including fluoride and bromide.

5. **They react to another ingredient or contaminant.** This can be true with any supplement, as it might not be the nutrient or herb someone is reacting to, but other ingredients or fillers. This is one of the downsides of taking kelp supplements, as while it's great that kelp is a food source of iodine, kelp supplements can be contaminated with heavy metals, and so it's possible that the person who has a negative effect when taking kelp isn't reacting to the iodine, but instead is reacting to the toxic metals. Of course if someone has a negative reaction with different forms of iodine then one can be more confident that they are reacting to the iodine, and not a different ingredient.

Iodine and Thyroid Nodules...What Does The Research Show?

I'll be discussing thyroid nodules in Chapter 21, but in this chapter I wanted to discuss what the research shows with regards to iodine and thyroid nodules. Some studies show that low iodine can be a factor in the development of thyroid nodules,[88, 89] but other studies show that too much iodine can also be a factor.[91, 92] So it really comes down to balance, as if you have one or more thyroid nodules it might be related to an iodine deficiency, but there is also a chance that excessive consumption of iodine is the culprit.

And as I'll discuss in Chapter 21, there are other factors which can lead to the development of thyroid nodules. This includes problems with estrogen metabolism and insulin resistance. And so in addition to considering an iodine imbalance as a cause of thyroid nodules you might also want to look into these factors.

Should Pregnant Women With Hyperthyroidism Supplement With Iodine?

There is no question that iodine is important to the developing fetus, as iodine deficiency during pregnancy can cause maternal and fetal hypothyroidism and impair neurological development of the fetus.[92] And so while anyone with hyperthyroidism will want to be cautious about supplementing with larger doses of iodine, I think it's a huge mistake to completely avoid iodine during pregnancy. And so I definitely recommend a prenatal with iodine to my pregnant patients with hyperthyroidism.

In summary, there is a lot of controversy involving iodine and hyperthyroidism. Although I personally had a positive experience with iodine supplementation when I was dealing with Graves' disease, and while I commonly recommended iodine testing and supplementation to my patients in the first few years of practice, I eventually realized that not everyone does well with iodine. Iodine has many benefits, as it is important for the production of thyroid hormone, it helps with the detoxification of halides, it has antimicrobial properties, it plays a role in estrogen metabolism, and it can help to prevent damage from radiation exposure.

However, there can be risks with iodine supplementation as well, as in some cases iodine can trigger thyroid autoimmunity, and it might induce hypothyroidism or hyperthyroidism in some individuals. Making sure someone has healthy antioxidant levels will reduce the risk of iodine triggering or exacerbating the autoimmune response, but I still would be cautious about taking separate iodine supplements.

Read The Following If You Choose To Supplement With Iodine

While you know that I'm cautious about iodine supplementation in those with hyperthyroidism, I realize that there will still be people who want to "experiment" with iodine. If you do this I would highly recommend for you to work with a natural healthcare practitioner. Chances are they will recommend testing for an iodine deficiency.

While there is no perfect test for measuring an iodine deficiency, without question some tests are better than others. Perhaps the least reliable method is through an Iodine Patch test. This test involves taking a 2% tincture of iodine, and essentially drawing a 2 x 2 "patch" on your forearm, stomach, or inner thigh with the iodine tincture.

If a person has a sufficient amount of iodine in their body, then the patch shouldn't begin to fade significantly until after 24 hours. If it fades in less than 24 hours then the person is said to have an iodine deficiency. If it fades in 12 hours or less then the person has a more severe iodine deficiency. Once again, this isn't the most accurate way of detecting an iodine deficiency, as just about everyone will have the patch fade in less than 24 hours, and the majority will have it fade in less than 12 hours.

Blood vs. Urine Testing

Blood testing for iodine is also highly unreliable. Urine testing seems to be the best method of testing, and there are a few different urine tests to choose from. One is a urinary spot test, which is a quick snapshot of current levels of Iodine in the body. A level below 0.15 mg/L is defined as an iodine deficient state according to the World Health Organization.

Another option is an iodine loading test. This is a urine test which measures the amount of iodine excreted over a 24-hour period. It involves taking a 50mg tablet of iodine/iodide, and then seeing how much is excreted through the urine over the next 24 hours. It's not the most convenient test, as you need to collect ALL of your urine within a 24 hour period, as just missing a single urine sample will make the results inaccurate.

If 90% of the ingested iodine/iodide is excreted, then the person supposedly has a sufficient amount of iodine. On the other hand, if they excrete less than 90% of iodine/iodide then they have an iodine deficiency.[93] So for example, a person who excretes only 20% of the iodine/iodide ingested is more iodine deficient than someone who excretes 50% of the iodine/iodide.

An elevated serum thyroglobulin can also be a sign of an iodine deficiency. In fact, numerous studies show that thyroglobulin can be used as a functional biomarker of iodine status.[94, 95, 96] I usually don't rely on this marker to determine if someone has an iodine deficiency, but some feel that thyroglobulin is a superior marker over urine because it reflects long-term iodine intake.

Some Research Studies Show That Iodine Can Help With Hyperthyroidism

While some people recommend for everyone with a hyperthyroid condition to completely avoid iodine, there is some evidence which shows that iodine can benefit those with hyperthyroidism. However, it's important to point out that these were older studies, and most involved consuming low amounts of iodine (i.e. from food sources). One study with the Danish population involving 8,219 people looked at the effect of higher iodine intake on thyroid hormone, and discovered that after the introduction of a mandatory iodization program it led to a lower prevalence of hyperthyroidism.[97]

Another study showed that patients with hyperthyroidism given 2mg or 4mg of iodine daily showed thyroid inhibition, and that "improvement was apparent within 48 hours".[98] So this is one study that did involve supplementing with decent amounts of iodine, but keep in mind that the study was from 1962. Yet another study showed that the benefits of correcting an iodine deficiency far outweigh the risks of iodine supplementation.[99]

Dr. David Brownstein has written a very interesting book called, "Iodine, Why You Need It, Why You Can't Live Without It". In his book Dr. Brownstein states the following: "The rising incidence of Hashimoto's and Graves' disease correlates with falling iodine levels." He also says "I believe the increase in both Hashimoto's and Graves' disease is due in large part to iodine deficiency."[100] I should also mention that in the book Dr. Brownstein discusses taking very large doses of iodine, and as you now know, not everyone does well with iodine supplementation.

That being said, the controversy over iodine supplementation most likely will continue. If you do enough research you can find studies which reveal that iodine can help people with hyperthyroidism and Graves' disease, like the ones I've included in this chapter. But other studies will show that iodine can be a potential trigger of hyperthyroidism and thyroid autoimmunity. There is no question that iodine is an important mineral, and while having any mineral deficiency isn't a good thing, you do want to be cautious when it comes to supplementing with iodine.

Chapter Summary

- Although I'm cautious about people with hyperthyroidism supplementing with iodine, I don't advise people to avoid all food sources of iodine, and I'm usually not concerned about iodine in a multivitamin
- While I no longer routinely advise patients with thyroid and autoimmune thyroid conditions to supplement with iodine, if you choose to do so you will want to make sure you have healthy levels of selenium
- 5 reasons why some people experience problems with iodine supplementation include 1) they don't have an iodine deficiency, 2) they are taking too large of a dose, 3) they have low levels of antioxidants, 4) they experience a "detox" reaction, and 5) they react to another ingredient or contaminant.
- I do recommend a prenatal with iodine to my pregnant patients with hyperthyroidism.

For access to the book references and resources, visit
savemythyroid.com/hyperbooknotes

CHAPTER 14

Can Environmental Toxins Trigger Graves' Disease?

IN THE SECOND EDITION of my book I mentioned the book called the Autoimmune Epidemic, which talks about how autoimmune conditions were on the rise, yet they still didn't gain the attention that cancer and heart disease have received. The author of the book, Donna Jackson Nakazawa, talks a great deal about how environmental toxins are potentially responsible for many of the autoimmune conditions which exist. Since then there have been other great books released related to the negative impact of environmental toxins, including The Toxin Solution by Dr. Joseph Pizzorno, and Dirty Girl: Ditch the Toxins, Look Great and Feel FREAKING AMAZING by Dr. Wendie Trubow and Dr. Ed Levitan.

There are over one hundred autoimmune conditions, and the bad news is that someone with Graves' disease is more likely to develop one or more additional autoimmune conditions when compared to the general public.

This makes sense when you think about it, as the factors I discussed in an earlier chapter which can trigger an autoimmune thyroid condition like Graves' disease can also trigger a different type of autoimmune condition.

Although I talk a great deal about how lifestyle factors and nutritional deficiencies can contribute to or directly cause an autoimmune thyroid condition, we can't discount the impact environmental toxins have on our health. After all, in this day and age we are being exposed to chemicals which weren't in existence decades ago. And so it is of no coincidence that as we are being exposed to more environmental toxins, the rate of autoimmune conditions is increasing. As Donna Jackson Nakazawa revealed in her book, companies aren't required to report whether these toxins can do harm to the immune system:

> *"While chemical companies have to divulge information if their chemicals have been found to be carcinogenic in lab testing, no such testing and reporting are required on whether chemicals act as autogens and damage the human immune system".*[101]

Even though her book was published in 2009, I'm pretty sure this is still true over a decade later. And it's not due to the lack of research, as there are many studies which show a relationship between different environmental toxins and autoimmunity.[102, 103, 104]

Be Careful About What You Bring Into Your Home

Unlike diet and lifestyle factors, you don't have complete control with regards to the environmental toxins you're exposed to on a daily basis. This is especially true when you step outside of your home. It is impossible to avoid all of the environmental toxins out there, but most people can do a better job of minimizing their exposure to them, and a lot can be done inside your own home. A big area is with the household products people buy, as this is a huge problem which exposes people to many of these toxins.

One of the primary toxins we're exposed to on a frequent basis is xenoestrogens. And when trying to restore one's health through a natural treatment approach, xenoestrogens are one of the main factors which can affect a person's recovery. While many people with thyroid and autoimmune thyroid conditions are aware they need to eat better, exercise more, and modify other lifestyle factors, most people don't pay enough attention to xenoestrogens, along with other endocrine-disrupting chemicals (EDCs). So what I'd like to do is briefly talk about what xenoestrogens are, how they affect your health, and what you can do to minimize your exposure to them.

Xenoestrogens are substances which contain synthetic estrogen, and therefore have a hormone-like effect on the body. Many of today's products and foods contain synthetic hormones, which without question have a profound effect on our endocrine systems, as well as our overall health. Some of the products and foods which contain xenohormones include:

- Pesticides
- Herbicides
- Fungicides
- Detergents
- Nail polish and nail polish remover
- Meat from livestock fed hormones to increase their size
- Many non-organic dairy products
- Many cosmetics
- Paint remover
- Some types of soaps
- Glues
- Most plastics (even BPA free)
- Many perfumes and air fresheners

While xenoestrogens can affect the health of anyone with a thyroid condition (as well as those people who don't have a thyroid disorder), people with an autoimmune thyroid disorder are arguably affected even more. So those people with Graves' disease need to take extra precautions in order to minimize their exposure to xenoestrogens, as they can have a negative effect on the immune system.

In fact, here is a quote from the book entitled "What Your Doctor May Not Tell You About Menopause", which was written by Dr. John R. Lee:

> *"More recent research is showing that exposure to xenohormones suppresses the immune-system, and in particular hampers T-lymphocyte function, and lowers the proportions and numbers of natural killer (NK) cells. These are two of your immune system's most important defenses. The latest studies are showing even more widespread damage to the immune system."*[105]

Other Harmful Effects Of Xenoestrogens

In addition to compromising one's immune system, there are many other side effects that xenoestrogens can have. Keep in mind that most of the time the effects aren't immediate, as it takes years for these symptoms and conditions to develop. But some of the different symptoms include fatigue, headaches, depression, lack of concentration, increased mood swings and irritability, and many other symptoms.

If this sounds similar to some of the side effects of a hormone imbalance, this is because xenoestrogens essentially disrupt the endocrine system, and therefore create a hormone imbalance. The reason for this is because they closely resemble our natural hormones, which allows them to bind to the same receptors. So for example, synthetic estrogens will bind to the estrogen receptors. But they don't have the same functions as natural estrogens, which is why they will cause many different side effects.

But they cause more than just side effects. As mentioned previously, exposure to these toxins can potentially lead to the development of an autoimmune condition. Research studies also show that long-term exposure to xenohormones can disrupt the gut microbiome[106] and can increase the incidence of certain types of cancers.[107] So hopefully you're beginning to realize how dangerous these toxins are, and will begin trying to do everything you can to minimize your exposure to them.

And if you are of childbearing age and are thinking of having children, keep in mind that studies also show that xenohormones can affect future generations.[108] So when a patient of mine informs me that she is trying to get pregnant, one of the things I'll recommend is for her to focus on reducing her toxic load prior to becoming pregnant to help eliminate some of the environmental toxins, including many of these xenoestrogens. This will help to put her in a better state of health before she becomes pregnant and help to minimize her babies' exposure to these toxins.

It is of course impossible to avoid all of the environmental toxins out there. However, as I have already mentioned, many of the xenoestrogens we're exposed to are a result of the foods and products we bring into our own homes, and so this is something we CAN control.

When you think about it, there is really no good reason to purchase products which contain potentially harmful chemicals. Especially when there are natural alternatives out there for most of these products. Sure, they will most likely cost more than the brand-name products most people buy, but it's definitely worth the extra money spent.

If you're not familiar with the Skin Deep database by the Environmental Working Group, I highly recommend checking it out, which you can do by visiting www.ewg.org/skindeep. As stated on their website, Skin Deep makes it easier for shoppers to understand potential hazards and health concerns related to ingredients in cosmetics and personal care products.

They compare the ingredients on personal care product labels and websites to the information in nearly 60 toxicity and regulatory databases. Then they give every product and ingredient in the database a two-part score—one for hazard and one for data availability.

Can Air Fresheners Cause Asthma?

Some of these chemicals shouldn't be used at all in my opinion. For example, I remember when growing up as a child my mother constantly would use air fresheners in our house. Just like most people, she didn't realize the potential damage these chemicals can cause to the lungs and other tissues in the body when used frequently. Perhaps it's no coincidence that she eventually developed asthma (although to be fair, she did smoke for many years as well, which obviously can be a big factor).

I'm not suggesting that everyone who uses air fresheners will develop asthma, or any other health condition for that matter. However, many people use similar chemicals in their home on a daily basis and assume that they are completely safe, but many of them aren't. There is a lot of evidence showing that certain consumer products include endocrine disrupters and asthma-associated chemicals.[109] This not only includes air fresheners, but perfumes, dryer sheets, and sunscreens.

The book "Dirty Girl: Ditch the Toxins, Look Great and Feel FREAKING AMAZING!" by Dr. Wendie Trubow goes beyond household products, and it's definitely a book that's worth reading. You can also listen to the interviews I did with Dr. Trubow on my podcast. The reason why I'm spending a lot of time focusing on household products is because this is a big area in which most people can control.

One of the main goals of this chapter is to make you aware that there are many things in our environment we don't think of as being toxic. I guarantee that most women don't think of the negative health consequences when they put on nail polish. And of course many parents put nail polish on their children's fingernails as well. Another thing to keep in mind is that some of these environmental chemicals might take years to cause or contribute to the development of an autoimmune condition, and of course not everyone develops a chronic health condition from exposure to these chemicals.

In fact, I think it's safe to say that most women won't develop Graves' disease just because they use nail polish. On the other hand, the combination of nail polish and other toxic cosmetics, household cleaners, and other products may very well increase their chances of developing Graves' disease or another autoimmune condition. And since problems with estrogen metabolism can be a factor in the development of toxic multinodular goiter, it's possible that endocrine-disrupting chemicals can also play a role in the development of this condition. The truth is we don't completely know the impact of these chemicals on our health, but as I mentioned before, since there are alternative options out there it makes sense to purchase products that are natural and try everything you can to avoid chemicals which can have a negative impact on your health.

The Effects Of Indoor and Outdoor Pollution On Thyroid Health

Many of the people I consult with have already made some great changes with their diet, and many also have incorporated other lifestyle changes, such as managing their stress. But most don't focus enough on minimizing their exposure to environmental toxins. I've already discussed the impact that household products can have on one's health, but now I want to take a little bit of time to talk about indoor and outdoor air pollution. Because even if you eat a perfect diet and buy all organic household products and cosmetics, you will still be exposed to thousands of chemicals in the air you breathe.

As part of my Masters in Nutrition degree I took a detoxification course, which was taught by Dr. Walter Crinnion. I spoke about Dr. Crinnion in an earlier chapter, as he was a naturopathic doctor who before passing away in 2019 had been in practice for about 30 years, and he focused on environmental pollution and detoxification. During the detoxification course Dr. Crinnion discussed some of the top sources of outdoor air pollution:

- Transportation: cars, buses, trucks
- Fuel consumption in stationary sources
- Industrial processes
- Forest fires
- Solid waste disposal
- Chemical dumps
- Aerial spraying of farms

As for some of the most common pollutants we're exposed to, these include volatile organic compounds (VOCs), which are solvents such as benzene and xylene. Other toxins we're commonly exposed to include Polycyclic aromatic hydrocarbons (PAH), carbon monoxide, ozone, heavy metals, pesticides, and herbicides.

As for indoor pollution, besides the chemicals associated with common household products and cosmetics, here are some of the other sources of toxins:

- Mothballs and deodorants (have paradichlorobenzene)
- Plastics, foam rubber, and insulation (styrene)
- Dry cleaning (contain tetrachloroethylene)
- Paints (styrene and xylene)
- Tap water(chloroform)
- Carpets (can contain VOCs, formaldehyde, dust mites, and other toxins)

How Do These Toxins Affect Thyroid Health?

There is a study which reveals the impact that numerous chemicals have on thyroid peroxidase (TPO) activity.[110] It shows that benzyophenones, PAHs, and persistent organic pollutants did slightly alter TPO activity at low doses. Some of the chemicals in this study decreased TPO activity, while others increased TPO activity. So when looking to restore the health of someone with hyperthyroidism or hypothyroidism, one can't overlook the impact of these toxins. I came across another study which shows that certain benzene-related compounds (they used 1-chloro-4-benzene and 1,3-diethyl benzene) can lead to thyroid dysfunction.[111]

There are also numerous studies involving pesticide exposure and thyroid disease. One study showed an increased risk of hypothyroidism with use of organochlorine insecticides and fungicides but no association with use of herbicides, fumigants, organophosphates, pyrethroids, or carbamates.[112]

Although some of these studies show that these chemicals inhibit thyroid function, thus leading to a hypothyroid condition, they also affect the immune system and can potentially trigger an autoimmune response. One study I came across showed evidence that organochlorine pesticides led to acceleration of autoimmunity.[113] Another study showed that tetrachloroethylene, which is found in dry cleaning, is associated with immunotoxicity.[114]

The Relationship Between Cigarette Smoking and Graves' Disease

A few different studies show that cigarette smoking can lead to the development of Graves' disease and Graves ophthalmopathy.[115, 116] I never smoked in my life, although my mother smoked in my home during my childhood and teenage years. I wasn't able to come across any evidence showing that secondhand smoke can cause Graves' disease, although one study showed that it might disrupt thyroid function, and might exacerbate thyroid autoimmunity.[117]

Heavy Metals Can Also Trigger An Autoimmune Response

In addition to the environmental toxins I've discussed thus far there are many others which can compromise our health. The next category I'd like to discuss is heavy metals, which includes mercury, aluminum, lead, cadmium, and arsenic. These toxic metals can without question have a profound impact on one's health, which is why I recommend that everyone does testing for heavy metals. I personally recommend a hair mineral analysis test, although some natural healthcare professionals will utilize provoked urine testing. Just keep in mind that no test is going to reveal all of the heavy metals in one's body, let alone other environmental toxins.

Mercury

There are numerous factors which can trigger an autoimmune response, and some of the heavy metals can cause this to happen as well. Mercury is one of the main heavy metal responsible for this.

Some of the more common sources of mercury exposure include dental amalgams, larger fish, vaccines, industrial use, and these days a lot of babies are being born with higher levels of mercury that are passed on from the mother. This of course is the case with other heavy metals as well, along with other toxins.

Even though mercury can potentially trigger an autoimmune response, the organ most affected by this heavy metal is the brain. In order to help to reduce your exposure to mercury you want to avoid eating larger fish, consider replacing dental amalgams, and try to avoid other sources. However, you need to be very cautious when getting dental amalgams removed, and if you do get this done I would highly recommend consulting with a biological dentist. A good resource for finding one is by going online and visiting the website for the International Academy of Oral Medicine and Toxicology (iaomt.org).

Aluminum

Some of the common sources of aluminum include pots and pans, aluminum cans, deodorant, aluminum foil, and some vaccines. Aluminum is another environmental toxin that can be found in tap water. Evidence suggests that high levels of aluminum can be a factor in the development of Alzheimer's disease.[118, 119]

Although I didn't find any research that showed a link between aluminum exposure and Graves' disease, keep in mind that aluminum is a demonstrated neurotoxin and a strong immune stimulator.[120] This is why aluminum is commonly added to vaccines as an adjuvant.

An adjuvant is a substance that is added to a vaccine to increase the body's immune response to the vaccine. Experimental evidence shows that simultaneous administration of as little as two to three immune adjuvants can overcome genetic resistance to autoimmunity.[121] In other words, even if you have a genetic resistance to developing autoimmune conditions such as Graves' disease, there is the possibility this condition can be triggered by exposure to multiple adjuvants.

Exposure to multiple adjuvants happens quite frequently in children through the routine administration of vaccinations. In some countries, by the time children are four to six years old, they will have received a total of 126 antigenic compounds along with high amounts of aluminum adjuvants through routine vaccinations.[122]

Arsenic

Some of the sources of arsenic include pesticides, herbicides, chicken, and brown rice. Exposure to arsenic in drinking water is common in many countries.[123] Inorganic arsenic is considered to be toxic. The highest levels of these arsenics in groundwater occur in the West, Midwest, and Northeast regions of the United States.

A journal article discussed how high concentrations of inorganic arsenic are found in some rice-based foods and drinks widely used in infants and young children.[124] Thus, while adults need to be cautious about consuming large amounts of inorganic arsenic, if you have children, then you want to make sure that they aren't eating large amounts of these foods. Poultry and seafood are the primary sources of organic arsenics, which are considered to have very low toxicity.

The health consequences of chronic arsenic exposure include increased risk for various forms of cancer and many noncancerous effects, including diabetes, skin diseases, chronic cough, and toxic effects on the liver, kidney, cardiovascular system, and peripheral and central nervous systems. While I couldn't find any research that shows a relationship between arsenic exposure and Graves' disease, evidence indicates that exposure to arsenic can directly affect thyroid health,[125] possibly by affecting the thyroid hormone receptors.[126]

Cadmium

Some of the sources of cadmium include cigarette smoke, tap water, coffee, shellfish, refined foods, and marijuana. Studies suggest that cadmium is associated with several clinical complications, such as renal dysfunction and bone disease, but also some cancers.[127] A few studies have shown that cadmium exposure can cause thyroid dysfunction.[128, 129] Just as mercury can potentially trigger autoimmunity, the same might be true of cadmium.[130]

Lead

Some of the common sources of lead exposure include cigarette smoke, colored inks, lead-based paints, ceramic glazes, and congenital causes. Diets deficient in calcium, magnesium, and/or iron can make someone more susceptible to a lead toxicity problem. Evidence indicates lead exposure can lead to depressed thyroid hormone levels.[131, 132] However, other studies show no relationship between lead exposure and thyroid health. It is possible that the amount of lead can play a role on how it affects thyroid health. While lead might play a role in autoimmunity,[133] I wasn't able to find any correlation in the research between lead and Graves' disease.

There are other toxic metals as well, although I'm not going to discuss them in great detail. Nickel is a toxic metal that can affect the brain and other organs of the body. Some of the other heavy metals include tin, uranium, thallium, and beryllium.

What Can You Do About These Environmental Toxins?

Okay, so now you know the impact that all of these environmental toxins can have on your health. So what can you do to 1) minimize your exposure to these toxins, and 2) eliminate them from your body? Here are some of the things to consider

- **Try to purchase as many natural household products as possible.** I realize this can be expensive, and if you can't afford to buy all natural products, then at the very least make sure those products you use on a frequent basis are natural. Earlier in this chapter I mentioned the Skin Deep database, which you can check out by visiting www.ewg.org/skindeep

- **Avoid drinking tap water and water from plastic bottles.** Occasionally drink tap water or water from plastic bottles isn't a big deal, but you don't want to drink from these sources on a consistent basis. I would recommend to either purify your water, or another option is to drink a good quality spring water from a glass bottle, such as Mountain Valley Springs.

- **Consider getting a chlorine filter for the shower, or consider investing in a whole house filter.** Many people drink purified water, but you absorb a good amount of chlorine when taking a five minute shower. So I would definitely consider getting a chlorine filter for your shower, and you might even want to think about getting a whole house filter.

- **If you have carpeting then consider replacing this.** I realize this might not be practical for many people, and if you're living in an apartment which has carpeting then this probably isn't an option. But there are a lot of chemicals present in carpet. In fact, according to the American Lung Association, carpets may trap pollutants and allergens like dust mites, pet dander, cockroach allergens, particle pollution, lead, mold spores, pesticides, dirt and dust.[134] Another option is to purchase carpeting made of natural ingredients. However, if you own your house I think hardwood floors are the best option, although keep in mind that the finish used for certain hardwood flooring can also emit toxins, such as formaldehyde. Fortunately you can purchase hardwood floors made with non-toxic adhesives and finishes.

- **If you dry clean your clothes, try to use a natural dry cleaning company (if available).** Tetrachloroethylene is used for most dry-cleaning fabrics, and is highly toxic.[135] In some areas this might not be an option, as there might not be a natural dry cleaning company nearby.

- **Be careful when purchasing new furniture.** This is due to the off-gassing. Just as is the case with carpeting, you can purchase "natural" furniture which doesn't have toxins. Even though the chemical emissions of furniture and carpeting are at the highest levels when these are brand new, they still emit toxins for many years, which is why it's a good idea to look into natural products, or consider purchasing used furniture.

- **Invest in a quality HEPA air purifier.** I personally have a few BlueAir purification systems (www.blueair.com), although there are other good companies which sell HEPA air purifiers. IQAir (www.iqair.com) is another great brand.

- **Change your HVAC filters regularly.** You not only want to change your HVAC filters regularly, but you also want to purchase high quality air filters.

- **Minimize your consumption of seafood.** This is controversial, as there are other natural healthcare practitioners who think it's fine to eat seafood on a daily basis, as long as you're avoiding larger fish. I think it's fine to eat some fish in moderation, and I agree that you want to try to minimize your consumption of the more toxic fish, such as swordfish, tuna, and halibut, and eat fish that are less toxic such as wild Alaskan salmon, flounder, whiting, and sardines.

- **If you have dental amalgams, consider getting them removed by a biological dentist.** This is somewhat controversial, as for example, if someone has a mouthful of silver fillings, and if they've had them for a long period of time, then depending on how they're removed it might do more harm than good. I realize that different natural healthcare professionals will have different opinions, as I know some who will recommend for all of their patients to get every single one of their silver fillings removed, and then will put them on chelation therapy for a few months. I think every situation is unique, and while it will benefit some people to get their silver fillings removed immediately, for others this might not be a wise decision. If you do choose to get them removed I definitely would recommend working with a biological dentist, and you can find one by visiting the website for the International Academy of Oral Medicine and Toxicology (www. iaomt.org).

- **Don't jog or cycle on a busy road.** There is evidence which shows that people who live in an urban environment and jog and/or cycle on a main road will have a greater toxic load. And this shouldn't be surprising, as when you think about all of the toxins emitted by cars, trucks, and buses, then you want to try engaging in aerobic exercise as far away as possible from these toxic sources.

- **Boost your glutathione levels.** I spoke about this in Chapter 12, as glutathione can help support the detoxification process. You can increase your glutathione levels by eating well, doing a good job of handling your stress, and minimizing your exposure to environmental toxins. You can also increase glutathione levels by eating cruciferous vegetables, and by supplementing with selenium, N-acetylcysteine, alpha lipoic acid, and/or milk thistle.

- **Look into other supplements which can help with detoxification, such as schisandra, burdock root, and dandelion.** I've already mentioned some supplements which can help with detoxification, but these are a few others that can help support detoxification.

- **Support the lymphatic system.** This is part of your immune system, and it has numerous functions, including maintaining body fluid levels and removing cellular waste. You can support lymphatic drainage simply through regular exercise, although some other methods include hot and cold showers, dry brushing, doing deep breathing, jumping rope, or rebounding.

- **Consider colon hydrotherapy and colonic irrigation.** Some people do need more extreme methods to help eliminate toxins. Colon hydrotherapy and colonic irrigation can effectively remove many of these toxins. However, you do want to make sure you see a certified colon hydrotherapist. Some people choose to do personal colon cleanses, including coffee enemas. These can help to eliminate toxins, but they're not as effective as colon hydrotherapy and colonic irrigation. However, doing colon cleanses at home, including coffee enemas, is a lot less expensive, and some people do benefit greatly from them. Coffee enemas can also help with liver detoxification by increasing glutathione production, and there are other potential benefits. Although coffee enemas aren't a part of my treatment recommendations for detoxification, I've had a few patients use coffee enemas prior to consulting with me, and most have reported positive results. If someone has problems with intestinal permeability it usually is a good idea to refrain from aggressive forms of colon cleansing.

- **Consider using an infrared sauna.** Using an infrared sauna is an excellent way to eliminate toxins from your body. Some healthcare professionals will recommend sauna therapy as their main treatment method for eliminating toxins. I definitely think sauna therapy can be beneficial, and I personally do sauna therapy two to three times per week, but you do want to make sure to take electrolytes to help replenish the lost nutrients. It's important to mention that if you have an uncontrolled elevated resting heart rate then you want to address this before doing sauna therapy.

In summary, the number of environmental toxins we've been exposed to over the years have increased dramatically, as has the number of autoimmune thyroid conditions such as Graves' disease. And while some might dismiss this as being a coincidence, books like "The Autoimmune Epidemic", "The Toxin Solution", "Dirty Girl", as well as others, show that environmental toxins do play a role in the increased incidence of these conditions. So hopefully this chapter motivates you to begin doing things to help reduce your toxic load.

Chapter Summary

- Although in this book I talk a great deal about how lifestyle factors and nutritional deficiencies can contribute to or directly cause an autoimmune thyroid condition, one can't discount the impact environmental toxins have.
- It is impossible to avoid all of the environmental toxins out there, but most people can do a better job of minimizing their exposure to them. Many of the toxins we're exposed to are cosmetics and other household products we buy.
- One of the primary toxins we're exposed to is xenoestrogens. Xenohormones are substances which contain synthetic hormones, primarily estrogen, and therefore have a hormone-like effect on the body.
- While xenoestrogens can affect the health of anyone with a thyroid condition (as well as those people who don't have a thyroid disorder), people with an autoimmune thyroid condition are arguably affected even more.
- Heavy metals such as mercury, aluminum, lead, cadmium, and arsenic can also compromise one's health.

For access to the book references and resources, visit
savemythyroid.com/hyperbooknotes

CHAPTER 15

The Role Of Infections In The Development Of Graves' Disease

ALTHOUGH MOST PEOPLE with Graves' disease have a genetic predisposition, by now you know that in order for autoimmunity to develop there needs to be an exposure to one or more environmental triggers. There are numerous factors which can trigger an autoimmune response. I've already discussed many of these factors in this book, as some of these factors include certain foods, chronic stress, and environmental toxins. But how about certain microbes? Numerous studies suggest that viruses, bacteria, and other microbes can lead to the development of an autoimmune condition.[136, 137]

But how do certain microbes specifically trigger an autoimmune response? I'm not going to get into too many specifics with regards to this, but essentially what happens is that the immune system responds by producing type 1 interferons and pro-inflammatory cytokines, which are directed at the microbe. In addition, something called pattern recognition receptors (PRR) are triggered, which recognize a large number of molecular patterns present in bacteria, viruses, and fungi.[138] This results in T-cell and B-cell activation,[138] and can ultimately result in an autoimmune response.

There is also the concept of molecular mimicry. What this essentially means is that some bacteria and viruses have amino acid sequences that are the same as humans. As a result, when a human is exposed to such a microbe, the immune system not only will attack the bacteria or virus, but since the microorganism has the same amino acid sequence as the human tissues, the immune system will also target the body tissues of the human, causing inflammation, and potentially triggering an autoimmune response. In addition, the virus or bacteria that triggers the autoimmune response may not be present by the time overt disease develops.[139]

Which Infections Can Lead To An Autoimmune Thyroid Condition?

There are numerous microorganisms which can potentially be a factor in the development of Graves' disease. I'm not going to list all of them here, but I'm going to talk about some of the more common ones.

Epstein-Barr Virus. Most people test positive for Epstein-Barr virus (EBV), but the good news is that it usually does not trigger an autoimmune response. With that being said, some studies have correlated EBV with Graves' disease.[140, 141] EBV is linked to infectious mononucleosis, and common symptoms include fever, sore throat, and swollen lymph glands. It is tested for through the blood, and while many natural healthcare practitioners will test for viral capsid antigen (VCA)-IgM, VCA-IgG, and Epstein Barr nuclear antigen (EBNA), perhaps the most important marker is Epstein-Barr early antigen (EBV-EA) IgG, which many don't test for. If the EBV-VCA IgM and/or EBV-EA IgG are elevated, this can indicate an active infection.

Cytomegalovirus. Cytomegalovirus is a type of herpes virus, and is related to the viruses that cause chickenpox and infectious mononucleosis. It is detected through the blood, and many people remain asymptomatic when they get infected with this virus. Most of the time treatment isn't necessary, although some doctors will prescribe antiviral medication.

Cytomegalovirus is linked to certain autoimmune conditions.[142] One study showed that cytomegalovirus, along with some other microbes, may be involved in the pathogenesis of Hashimoto's thyroiditis and Graves' disease.[143] I also came across a separate study which linked Graves' disease to this virus.[144]

Hepatitis C. Hepatitis C is a virus which can cause inflammation of the liver. This is transmitted through the blood, and some of the symptoms include abdominal pain and swelling, pale stools, dark urine, fatigue, fever, and jaundice.[145] Hepatitis C is usually detected through the blood, and conventional treatment methods consist of antiviral drugs. I came across one study which showed that Hepatitis C can lead to the development of Graves' disease.[146]

Yersinia enterocolitica. Yersinia enterocolitica is a bacteria that can lead to numerous health problems, such as enterocolitis, acute diarrhea, and pseudoappendicitis. The best way to test for this is through the stool. Conventional medical treatment consists of certain medications, such as aminoglycosides and tetracyclines. There is evidence that Yersinia enterocolitica might play a role in the pathogenesis of Graves' disease.[147, 148, 149]

H. Pylori. This is a bacteria located in the stomach, and numerous studies link H. Pylori with Graves' disease.[150, 151] H. Pylori can interfere with the production of stomach acid, which in turn will cause problems with digestion, and can also lead to bacterial and/or yeast overgrowth. There are numerous methods of testing for H. Pylori, with the urea breath test and stool antigen test the most common methods used by practitioners, although more recently there have been newer tests such as the GI-MAP, which utilizes quantitative PCR. This is supposed to increase the sensitivity and specificity of the test, and the lab also looks at the H. pylori virulence factors and antibiotic resistance genes.

Lyme Disease. Lyme disease is caused by a bacteria known as Borrelia burgdorferi, and is usually transmitted through the bite of a tick, and possibly through fleas as well. There is some evidence that Borrelia burgdorferi may be involved in the pathogenesis of autoimmune thyroid disease.[152] In 2018 I was diagnosed with chronic Lyme disease, but thankfully it didn't result in a relapse of my Graves' disease condition.

Testing For Infections

Different microorganisms will require different types of tests. For example, Lyme disease, Hepatitis C, Epstein Barr Virus, cytomegalovirus, and Yersinia enterocolitica are usually detected in the blood. On the other hand, stool testing can also help to determine Yersinia enterocolitica. As I mentioned earlier, there are numerous methods of testing for H. Pylori, as it could be tested through the blood, saliva, stool, and there is also a urea breath test. The problem with blood and saliva is that these are testing for the antibodies of H. pylori, and just because someone has positive antibodies doesn't mean that they have H. pylori.

Let's take a look at some of the tests that can detect infections:

Comprehensive stool panel. While a basic stool panel conducted at a local lab will look for acute gut pathogens (viruses, bacteria, and parasites that can cause gastroenteritis), there are a lot of things they don't test for. For example, they don't test for H. pylori, other types of parasites, opportunistic bacteria, commensal flora, markers of gut inflammation, etc. Some of the companies I recommended back when I wrote the second edition of this book are no longer in business, and so rather than list the ones I currently use here, I'll include them in the suggested resources, which you can check out by visiting savemythyroid.com/hyperbooknotes

Candida overgrowth. Although most comprehensive stool panels test for yeast, it's not the best test for a yeast overgrowth. I prefer an organic acids test (OAT), which isn't specific for yeast, as it also includes markers related to some of the nutrients, neurotransmitters, mitochondria, and indicators of detoxification. That being said, I usually won't recommend an OAT just to see if someone has a yeast overgrowth, and there are times when it will show up on a comprehensive stool panel. And so if you choose to do a comprehensive stool panel it makes sense to see if it picks up yeast, but if it doesn't just keep in mind that this doesn't rule out a yeast overgrowth.

Stealth infections. As I mentioned earlier, in 2018 I was diagnosed with chronic Lyme disease, along with bartonella. While you can test these at a local lab, false negatives are quite common, and so if you suspect you have a stealth infection you might want to choose a specialty lab, and I'll make sure to give a few options in the resources. I'll add that not everyone with stealth infections will have the classic symptoms.

This actually described me back in 2018, as I didn't have the classic symptoms associated with Lyme disease, and there was no evidence of a tick bite, no bulls eye rash. In fact, when I went to a primary care doctor he refused to test me for Lyme disease and wanted to refer me to a neurologist. At the time I wasn't 100% certain I had Lyme disease, but I strongly suspected I had it, and so I ended up consulting with a local Lyme specialist who practices functional medicine, and she did test me for Lyme disease through a specialty lab, which came back positive for chronic Lyme disease and bartonella.

Viruses. While some specialty labs also offer testing for viruses, including the one I used for my Lyme disease diagnosis, it's also fine to test for these through a local lab. This includes Epstein-Barr, Cytomegalovirus, Hepatitis C, and others I didn't list in this chapter, including Parvovirus B19 and herpes simplex.

Small intestinal bacterial overgrowth (SIBO). Currently the only way to test for SIBO is through a breath test. With the breath test the patient fasts overnight, and then in the morning they will start with a baseline breath sample, followed by the consumption of a substrate (i.e. lactulose or glucose). After the baseline breath sample they will measure a breath sample approximately every 20 minutes, and what the lab is looking for is bacterial fermentation, and it measures this fermentation by measuring the levels of hydrogen and methane. In other words, if someone has SIBO, there will be more fermentation, which will lead to higher levels of hydrogen, methane, or both gases. I should add that as of writing the third edition of this book there is a newer lab that tests for hydrogen, methane, and hydrogen sulfide.

How Can You Eradicate These Microbes?

If someone tests positive for any of these microorganisms, then how can they be eradicated? It can be challenging, and in many cases they can't be completely eradicated. For example, while an infection such as H. Pylori can be eradicated, if someone has a virus such as Epstein-Barr, or if they have Borrelia burgdorferi, which once again is the pathogen associated with Lyme disease, then these microorganisms cannot be completely eradicated.

In these cases the goal is to put them in a dormant state, and to help the person maintain their health so that they don't cause any problems.

Although different infections might require different protocols, having a healthy immune system is also very important, which I'll expand on towards the end of this chapter. But I'll say here that anything that compromises the health of your immune system (i.e. poor diet, chronic stress, lack of sleep), can make someone more susceptible to developing an infection. And so in many cases it's more of an immune problem than an infection problem.

Antimicrobial Supplements and Herbs

Some of the supplements and herbs which can help with numerous microbes include the following:

Goldenseal. This herb is used to help with inflammation and infection. Its antibacterial activity has been attributed to its alkaloids, the most abundant which is berberine.[153] Several studies demonstrate how effective berberine is when it comes to certain infections.[154, 155] In fact, over the last few years I've used berberine more than goldenseal. I should add that berberine doesn't just have antimicrobial properties, as it also can help with blood sugar imbalances (i.e. insulin resistance), and I'll also discuss how it can benefit people with thyroid eye disease in Chapter 22.

Oregano oil. Oregano oil can also help to eradicate certain microbes, including fungi such as Candida[156, 157] as well as parasites.[158] However, it can be harsh on the gut microbiome, as it also can have a negative effect on the beneficial microbes of the gut. This doesn't mean that I never use oregano oil, but you want to be careful about taking very large doses for a prolonged period of time.

Garlic. Many people are aware that garlic has antimicrobial properties, and this is also backed up in the research.[159] Numerous studies show that garlic can help with H. pylori.[160, 161] But garlic is also effective against other pathogens, and can be effective against those strains that have become resistant to antibiotics.[161] Garlic can be effective with both gram-negative and gram-positive bacteria.[162] And the good news is that it doesn't seem to harm the beneficial microbes of the gastrointestinal tract.

Mastic Gum. Numerous studies have shown that mastic gum can help to eradicate H. Pylori.[163, 164]

Cat's Claw (Uncaria tomentosa). Cat's Claw has immunomodulating, antimicrobial, and antiviral activities.[165, 166]

Probiotics. Probiotics can also play an important role in preventing and eradicating infections. Lactobacilli and bifidobacteria are most commonly found in probiotic supplements, but Saccharomyces boulardii can also help to eradicate certain microbes, such as Clostridium difficile[167] and can also help with yeast overgrowth.[168, 169] The research also shows that it can help with certain protozoa infections, including amebiasis, giardiasis and infection with Blastocystis hominis.[170, 171]

Caprylic Acid. Caprylic Acid also has antimicrobial properties,[172] especially against Streptococcus agalactiae, Streptococcus dysgalactiae, and Streptococcus uberis.[173] However, this can also be effective against other microbes.[174]

Pau D' Arco (Tabebuia avellanedae). For many decades, preparations made with this plant were used in South and North America as antineoplasic, antifungal, antiviral, antimicrobial, antiparasitic and antiinflammatory treatment.[175]

Colloidal Silver. Colloidal silver is commonly used as an antimicrobial, although there is some controversy over this. One study showed evidence that colloidal silver is a broad-spectrum antimicrobial agent against aerobic and anaerobic bacteria,[176] while another study showed that colloidal silver didn't have any antimicrobial effect in vitro on certain microorganisms.[177] I have had success with colloidal silver in my practice.

Wormwood (Artemisia absinthium). Wormwood is commonly used by natural healthcare professionals in the treatment of parasites.[178, 179]

Quercetin. Quercetin is a naturally occurring flavonoid, and evidence indicates that quercetin has antiviral activity against EBV.[180]

Olive Leaf. This is an herb that has antiviral properties,[181, 182] and one study showed that it has antibacterial activity against different H. pylori strains.[183]

As I mentioned before, some of these microorganisms can be very challenging to eradicate. For example, one of the more common bacteria I come across in my practice is H. Pylori. And while taking a natural treatment approach can frequently help people with this bacteria, it usually takes a couple of months to accomplish this. And sometimes the natural treatment methods aren't potent enough to eradicate H. Pylori, which means that the person might need to take antibiotics, which of course will further compromise the gut flora. Lyme disease is another pathogen that is difficult to manage, and unlike H. Pylori, the goal isn't necessarily to eradicate the infection, but instead the goal is to put it in a dormant state.

Taking a Conservative Approach vs. Using Antimicrobials

After reading this chapter you might be ready to test for infections and do whatever is necessary to eradicate them. And this is the approach I've taken for many years. But there is an argument for taking a more conservative approach in certain situations. For example, while I've interviewed practitioners on my podcast who will treat everyone for parasites, there are other natural healthcare practitioners who won't treat everyone for parasites...even if they were to test positive for parasites on a stool test. And the same thing goes for H. pylori, as while this can potentially be an autoimmune trigger, this isn't always the case.

So while for years my approach has been to put someone on an antimicrobial protocol if they test positive for H. pylori or parasites, another option is to take a more conservative approach. Now I do consider the use of natural agents to be more conservative than prescription drugs, but they can still cost a lot of money, and they don't always work. In other words, you might take natural antimicrobials for H. pylori or parasites for a few months, and upon retesting they might still come back positive.

While you can take certain supplements and herbs directed at these different microbes, perhaps the most important factor is to do things to improve the health of your immune system. This by far is the best method of maintaining your health. After all, we're all going to be exposed to certain microbes. But if you have a healthy immune system then this will minimize your chances of it becoming an infection. This isn't always going to be the case, as I felt like I had a healthy immune system and still ended up with chronic Lyme disease. However, at the time my symptoms weren't as bad as many others who have Lyme disease, and I think the reason for this is because over the years I had been doing a lot to optimize my immune system health.

It's also worth mentioning that certain foods can have antimicrobial properties. For example, in addition to doing things to improve your immune system health, eating garlic and fermented foods can help to prevent certain infections from developing. And having a healthy gut microbiome will also help minimize the potential negative impact that certain bacteria and parasites can have on your health.

In summary, certain microbes can potentially trigger an autoimmune response, thus leading to the development of a condition such as Graves' disease. And while natural treatment methods can frequently benefit people with these infections, it can be a challenge to restore someone's health when it's caused by a virus, bacteria, or another type of microorganism.

Chapter Summary

- Numerous studies suggest that viruses, bacteria, and parasites can lead to the development of an autoimmune condition
- Some pathogens which can potentially trigger an autoimmune thyroid condition include 1) Lyme Disease, 2) Hepatitis C, 3) Yersinia enterocolitica, 4) H. Pylori, 5) Epstein Barr Virus, and 6) Cytomegalovirus
- Detecting different microbes will require different types of tests, as some are best detected in the blood, while others are best detected in the stool.
- Some of the supplements and herbs which can help to eradicate microbes include 1) Goldenseal, 2) Oregano oil, 3) Garlic, 4) Mastic gum, 5) Cat's Claw, 6) Probiotics, 7) Caprylic acid, 8) Pau D' Arco, 9) Colloidal silver, 10) Wormwood, 11) Quercetin, and 12) Olive Leaf.

For access to the book references and resources, visit
savemythyroid.com/hyperbooknotes

CHAPTER 16

How Big Of A Role Does Genetics Play?

I'M SURE MANY PEOPLE with hyperthyroidism and Graves' disease wonder whether genetic factors played a major role in the development of their condition. In fact, I've had numerous patients ask me as to whether genetics is the primary reason why they have developed a thyroid or auto-immune thyroid condition, and whether this would prevent them from receiving good results when taking a natural treatment approach.

The truth is that many people with thyroid conditions have genetic markers which will make them more susceptible to developing such a condition. However, the research clearly shows that just because some-one has a genetic predisposition for a thyroid or autoimmune thyroid condition does not necessarily mean they will develop such a disorder. Although genetic factors do play a role, more and more studies are showing that lifestyle and environmental factors play an even greater role. In fact, Donna Jackson Nakazawa, the author of The Autoimmune Epidemic, also reveals the following:

"Twin studies show that autoimmune disease is roughly 30 percent genetic and 70 percent environmental. While two identical twins might hold the same genetic code for a certain autoimmune disease, either one of them will be struck with disease only if they meet up with the right environmental hit. As one researcher put it, while genetics may load the gun, it's environment that pulls the trigger."[184]

So even if you happen to have a genetic predisposition for Graves' disease, this does not mean you will develop this condition. And if you already have Graves' disease, you can still restore your health by taking a natural treatment approach, even if you do have a genetic predisposition.

This obviously is good news, as while some people might have an increased chance of developing hyperthyroidism or Graves' disease due to genetic factors, most of these people who don't have a such a condition can take steps to prevent such a disorder from developing. And as I've already mentioned, those people who do have an existing hyperthyroid condition can potentially restore their health by taking a natural treatment approach, despite having a genetic predisposition for such a disorder.

Other Resources Show That Lifestyle Factors Play An Important Role

Obviously I don't expect anyone to simply take my word for it that lifestyle factors play an equally important role, and perhaps an even greater role than genetics in determining whether or not someone develops a thyroid or autoimmune thyroid condition. I've already listed some resources which show that this is true. But if you want to read more about this, there are a few books out there that will discuss the importance of lifestyle factors when it comes to developing certain conditions.

One book is called "Outsmart Your Genes: How Understanding Your DNA Will Empower You to Protect Yourself Against Cancer, Alzheimer's, Heart Disease, Obesity, and Many Other Conditions", which is written Dr. Brandon Colby, and he goes into detail about genetics and predictive medicine, and how using genetic testing can help to prevent the development of certain conditions, including thyroid disorders. Another book, called the "Biology of Belief", by Bruce Lipton , also talks about genetics and how genes and DNA aren't the sole factors when it comes to developing certain conditions.

Just keep in mind that these books aren't specific to thyroid conditions. For example, in the book "Outsmart Your Genes", Dr. Colby talks about some of the different conditions which are determined by a combination of genetic and nongenetic factors. In addition to thyroid conditions, other examples of such conditions include heart disease, cancer, Parkinson's, Alzheimer's, and arthritis. Without question, there are certain diseases which are solely determined by genetics, and aren't influenced by lifestyle factors. Some examples include Tay-Sachs disease and cystic fibrosis. While there might not be much we can do to prevent or cure a disease such as cystic fibrosis, many of these other conditions can be prevented or in some cases completely cured.

Epigenetics and Thyroid Autoimmunity

The books I just mentioned were included in the first two editions of this book, and I decided to leave them in this third edition because they are still relevant. But I figured I'd also share some of the research that shows how environmental factors play a bigger role than genetics when it comes to the development of autoimmune conditions such as Graves' disease.

By the way, epigenetics involves changes in gene expression that doesn't affect the DNA sequence.

One journal article discussed the epigenetic mechanism for discordance of autoimmunity in identical twins,[185] who share an identical DNA sequence. Because of this, if genetics was the only factor in the development of autoimmunity then you'd figure that if one identical twin developed an autoimmune condition, that the second one would develop it as well, but this definitely isn't the case. Another journal article showed that epigenetic pathways play a pivotal role in the development and function of the immune system,[186] and another journal article mentioned that the environment can contribute to autoimmunity by modifying gene expression through epigenetic mechanisms.[187]

Does Having A Genetic Predisposition Mean You're More Likely To Experience A Relapse?

As I have already mentioned numerous times, people with a genetic marker for a hyperthyroid condition can restore their health through a natural treatment approach. However, you might wonder if having a genetic predisposition means you are more likely to experience a relapse after restoring your health. I don't know if there is a specific answer to this, but my response is "probably so". The reason is because while a person with hyperthyroidism can restore their health, if they also have a genetic marker for this condition, and then goes on to neglect those lifestyle factors I have discussed in this book, then there is a good chance they will suffer a relapse over time.

However, this might also hold true for those people who don't have a genetic predisposition for a thyroid or autoimmune thyroid condition. In other words, if someone without a genetic marker develops a thyroid condition solely due to lifestyle factors, restores their health through natural treatment methods, and then neglects their health again, then there is a good chance they will suffer a relapse.

This is yet another reason why I don't like to use the word "cure", as my goal is not to cure any condition, but rather is to help the person achieve optimal health and then show them how to maintain a state of wellness. I of course spoke about this in detail in Chapter 6, talking about the difference between a permanent cure and a state of remission. Either way, one needs to maintain their health or there is a chance their condition can return.

As you know, I've been in remission from Graves' disease since 2009. So as of writing the third edition of this book it's been almost 14 years, which I'm very grateful for. But this doesn't mean that I can never relapse, and so while I'm not perfect with my diet and lifestyle, I still do a lot to maintain a state of wellness.

So while there is always a chance for a relapse to occur whether someone has a genetic predisposition or not, if you do restore your health and then maintain a state of wellness, then this will obviously decrease the chances of you suffering a relapse. In summary, genetics without question can be a factor in developing a thyroid or autoimmune thyroid condition, but it isn't the only factor. Lifestyle and environmental factors at least play an equally important role, and there is a lot of evidence which shows that these factors are probably more important than genetics.

Chapter Summary

- Research shows that just because someone has a genetic marker for a thyroid or autoimmune thyroid condition does not necessarily mean they will develop such a disorder.
- Lifestyle and environmental factors can play a greater role in determining whether someone will develop a thyroid or autoimmune thyroid disorder.
- Because genetics is a factor there is always a chance that someone with a thyroid or autoimmune thyroid condition can relapse after restoring their health, which is why I choose not to use the word "cure", but instead strive to help people achieve a state of "permanent remission".

For access to the book references and resources, visit
savemythyroid.com/hyperbooknotes

CHAPTER 17

Graves' Disease & Thyroid Antibodies

POSITIVE THYROID STIMULATING immunoglobulins (TSI) means that someone has the autoimmune component associated with Graves' disease. This is true even if other thyroid blood tests are negative, as it's important to understand that with Grave' disease, the autoimmune response will develop first, and will then be followed by malfunctioning of the thyroid gland.

This might seem to be confusing to those people with Graves' disease who consider their condition to be a thyroid condition. Graves' disease is really an autoimmune condition which leads to thyroid malfunction. In other words, the malfunctioning thyroid gland is usually not the actual cause of the disorder in an autoimmune thyroid condition, as I have already discussed in other chapters.

So while most people with Graves' disease have a low TSH and/or high thyroid hormone levels, one can be positive for thyroid antibodies without having these other blood tests positive. How does this process develop? Elaine Moore does a wonderful job of discussing the different types of antibodies in her book "Graves Disease, A Practical Guide". She discusses how the "TSI acts as an agonist, mimicking TSH and causing excess thyroid hormone production".[188]

So this antibody will cause an excess of thyroid hormone by binding to or stimulating the TSH receptors, which eventually will lead to the low TSH and high free T3 and T4 levels. She also discusses the thyroid growth stimulating immunoglobulins (TGI), and states that "when Graves' disease patients are tested for both TGI and TSI, nearly 100 percent of patients are positive for one or the other antibody".[189]

Although there are a few older studies showing the presence of TGI in those with Graves' disease, these aren't commonly tested for by endocrinologists. One reason is because not all labs offer this test. And I'll say here that I have relied on the TSI over the years, although some doctors will test for the thyrotropin receptor antibodies (TRAB), which is also fine.

Many people with Graves' disease also have positive thyroid peroxidase (TPO) antibodies. These confirm the presence of an autoimmune thyroid condition, but they aren't specific to Graves' disease, as most people with Hashimoto's thyroiditis will also have elevated TPO antibodies. Regardless of the type of thyroid antibodies you have, the obvious goal will be to restore the health of your immune system so that all of these antibodies will eventually be negative. This admittedly can be challenging at times, and it all comes down to finding and removing your triggers and correcting any underlying imbalances.

What Determines Which Autoimmune Thyroid Condition One Will Develop?

Why do some people develop Graves' disease, while other people develop Hashimoto's thyroiditis? It's a matter of having different antibodies, as this relates to the immune system affecting different parts of the thyroid gland. Genetics of course is a factor as to which thyroid antibodies a person will develop. If someone has a genetic predisposition for Graves' disease then they are more likely to develop thyroid stimulating immunoglobulins.

On the other hand, if they have a genetic predisposition towards Hashimoto's thyroiditis they are likely to develop TPO and/or anti-thyroglobulin antibodies, although many people with Graves' disease also have TPO antibodies. Of course this assumes something triggers the genetics, as I have already discussed in this book that just having a genetic predisposition for Graves' disease or any other condition doesn't mean you will develop that condition. It's also worth mentioning that it's not uncommon for people to have all three of the thyroid antibodies I mentioned (thyroid stimulating immunoglobulins, thyroid peroxidase antibodies, anti-thyroglobulin antibodies).

While I'm sure in the future we will discover even more about autoimmune thyroid conditions, what's important to understand for now is that in order to restore the health of anyone who has an autoimmune condition, you need to do more than manage the symptoms. This is where conventional medicine fails, as most conventional medical treatments are aimed at managing the symptoms of the autoimmune condition, as you have learned in this book. This isn't just the case with Graves' disease, but with many other autoimmune conditions as well. For example, someone with Hashimoto's thyroiditis will almost always be told to take synthetic or desiccated thyroid hormone, but nothing will be done to address the autoimmune response. So the person will take thyroid hormone replacement daily to help with the symptoms while their thyroid gland continues to be damaged by the immune system.

It's a similar situation with Graves' disease, as when I was initially diagnosed by my endocrinologist, she recommended antithyroid drugs, along with a beta blocker to manage my symptoms. And while she didn't talk much about radioactive iodine treatment, there is little doubt that if I decided to take the antithyroid drugs and if they failed to put my condition into remission, then RAI probably would have been brought up as the "solution". But nothing was ever mentioned by her as to how I should restore the health of my immune system, adrenal glands, and other compromised areas of my body, and this is how most endocrinologists and other types of medical doctors think. Most don't try to do anything to address the cause of the condition, but are trained to simply manage the symptoms.

False Negatives Are Possible With Thyroid Antibodies

It's also important to know that someone with an autoimmune thyroid condition such as Graves' disease won't always have positive thyroid antibodies present on a blood test. So if you had a thyroid antibodies test and it came out negative, this doesn't confirm that you don't have an autoimmune condition. This is why it's important to also consider the patient's symptoms, other thyroid blood tests (although once again these might be negative as well), along with doing a thyroid ultrasound.

Because of this, if someone with Graves' disease takes a natural treatment approach, how do they know if they have had their health restored? In other words, if they initially had positive thyroid antibodies, but after a few months of taking a natural treatment approach they have a negative thyroid antibodies test, how can one be sure if their health has been restored, or if it's just a false negative? The answer is that you can't confirm that someone has had their health restored just by looking at the levels of thyroid antibodies once or twice.

I'll add that if someone with Graves' disease has tested positive for thyroid stimulating immunoglobulins then in most cases they will continue to test positive for these antibodies in the future until their immune system is balanced. And so in my experience it is rare to have someone test positive for TSI, and then a few months later test negative, and then a few months later test positive for them again. So even though the antibodies can fluctuate, it usually is a good sign when an antibodies test which was initially high continues to decrease over time.

However, if someone takes a natural treatment approach and their thyroid antibodies test comes out negative a single time then this doesn't confirm the autoimmune component has been permanently suppressed. Ideally I want to see this value negative for a least three consecutive readings a couple of months apart before coming to this conclusion. In addition, it's important to look at other factors, including the person's TSH and thyroid hormone levels, other tests that might have been recommended (adrenal testing, positive findings on a comprehensive stool test, hair mineral analysis, etc.), and of course their symptoms should be gone or at least greatly improved.

Some people reading this are familiar with the Th1 and Th2 pathways. Each of these pathways consists of different cytokines. The Th1 pathway consists of T-Helper cells which include the cytokines IL-2, IFN-γ, and tumor necrosis factor-α (TNF-α).[190] The Th2 pathway consists of B cells, and is characterized by the secretion of IL-4, IL-5, IL-6, IL-10, and IL-13.[190] Th1 cytokines are commonly found in Hashimoto's thyroiditis,[191] and thus Hashimoto's is typically known as a Th1-dominant condition. Graves' disease is thought to be a Th2-dominant autoimmune condition.[192] There is also a Th3 and Th17 pathway.

When I wrote the second edition of this book it was common for natural healthcare practitioners to focus on balancing the Th1 and Th2 pathways. In other words, they would do a blood test to see if their patient is Th1 or Th2 dominant, and then would give specific supplements or herbs depending on whether the person was Th1 or Th2 dominant. For example, if someone was Th1 dominant, they would recommend specific supplements and/or herbs to help stimulate the Th2 pathway. Similarly, if someone had a Th2-dominant condition they will do things in an attempt to stimulate the Th1 pathway. The problem is that this approach has flaws and shouldn't be relied upon, which is why only a small percentage of practitioners take this approach.

So based on what I've discussed so far, how does someone who is diagnosed with hyperthyroidism but has tested negative for thyroid stimulating immunoglobulins know for sure they don't have Graves' disease? According to some medical doctors this can confirmed through a radioactive iodine uptake test, which I'm about to discuss.

What You Need To Know About The Radioactive Iodine Uptake Test

Many people with hyperthyroidism receive a test called the radioactive iodine uptake test. With this test the patient swallows a small dose of radioactive iodine. Since the thyroid gland uses iodine to produce thyroid hormone, it will absorb the small dose of radioactive iodine. The absorption of the radioactive iodine is evaluated after six hours, and then again after 24 hours.

If the uptake of radioiodine is high then this indicates that your thyroid gland is producing an excess of thyroxine. This is usually due to Graves' disease, but in some cases it can also be related to thyroid nodules. If your radioiodine uptake test is low, but it's confirmed that you have hyperthyroidism, then you probably have thyroiditis. So the radioactive iodine uptake test doesn't offer 100% confirmation that someone has Graves' disease, although this test can give the medical doctor a better idea as to whether a person has this condition.

Will The Radioactive Iodine Uptake Test Damage Your Thyroid Gland?

I have received some emails from people who didn't want to receive this test because they were afraid it would damage their thyroid gland. Part of this is probably due to the fact that I frequently talk about the risks of radioactive iodine treatment, and how one should avoid this treatment method if at all possible.

But it's important to understand that the dose given for the radioactive iodine uptake test is much smaller than the dose given during radioactive iodine treatment. So does this mean that it's completely harmless to the thyroid gland? Well, any procedure which involves radiation isn't completely harmless, even if the dose is small. But this test most likely won't destroy enough thyroid cells to have a significant impact on thyroid function.

So should everyone with hyperthyroidism receive the radioactive iodine uptake test in order to confirm or rule out Graves' disease? I wouldn't necessarily recommend this, as if someone tests positive for hyperthyroidism and also has elevated thyroid stimulating immunoglobulins, then in my opinion it's usually not necessary to receive this test. On the other hand, if the TSI is negative, then obtaining the radioactive iodine uptake test can possibly help to determine if someone has Graves' disease.

After all, just because someone has a negative test for thyroid antibodies doesn't completely rule out Graves' disease, as I have already discussed.

And so if someone has negative thyroid stimulating immunoglobulins then perhaps they should consider getting the radioactive iodine uptake test. On the other hand, for someone who is looking to receive conventional medical treatment, receiving this test probably won't make much of a difference with regards to the treatment recommendations.

If you have hyperthyroidism, in most cases you will be told to take anti-thyroid drugs or receive RAI or surgery regardless of whether you have a positive or negative radioactive iodine uptake test. And this isn't just based on my opinion, as some studies suggest that the radioactive iodine uptake test doesn't do much when it comes to predicting the outcome of certain conventional treatment methods, such as RAI.[193] Although it can determine if someone has thyroid nodules, this can also be determined through an ultrasound, which is less invasive than a radioactive iodine uptake test.

That being said, some doctors will recommend the radioactive iodine uptake test to determine if someone has "hot" or "cold" nodules. If someone has a "cold" nodule there is a slightly greater increase in the thyroid nodule being malignant. However, it won't confirm or rule out a malignancy, and an ultrasound can also give an idea as to whether a thyroid nodule has a greater chance of being malignant based on certain characteristics (i.e. the size, if it's solid and/or has microcalcifications). I'll talk more about the characteristics of thyroid nodules in Chapter 21.

Contraindications Of This Test

Women who are pregnant or breastfeeding shouldn't receive the radioactive iodine uptake test.[194] The reason is because while the small dose of radioactive iodine isn't enough to cause harm to an adult, it can cause problems with a fetus or baby. If you're not sure whether or not you are pregnant, but suspect you might be, then it's best to hold off on this test.

It's also important to mention that thyroid eye disease is common in those with Graves' disease. As a result, if someone has hyperthyroidism and tests negative for the TSI, yet they have thyroid eye disease, then in all likelihood they have Graves' disease. That being said, just because you experience eye symptoms doesn't mean it's related to thyroid eye disease, and so you probably would want to visit an ophthalmologist to confirm this. I will discuss thyroid eye disease in greater detail in Chapter 22.

To summarize this chapter, the presence of thyroid antibodies is confirmation for an autoimmune thyroid condition. Thyroid stimulating immunoglobulins specifically confirm the presence of Graves' disease. On the other hand, a negative test for thyroid antibodies doesn't completely rule out Graves' disease. For someone with positive antibodies, it shouldn't come to a surprise that taking a natural treatment approach may result in future negative tests for thyroid antibodies. Even though one can't rely on the presence or absence of these levels, it still is a good feeling when someone has had multiple tests for thyroid antibodies, all of which were positive, and then to see these same tests come out negative after taking a natural treatment approach.

As for the radioactive iodine uptake test, although this treatment method won't obliterate the thyroid gland, it still does involve a small dose of radiation. As a result, while receiving this test shouldn't cause much harm to the thyroid gland, because it does involve some radiation I wouldn't recommend for everyone with hyperthyroidism to receive it. The question you need to ask yourself is "will receiving this test affect the course of treatment?" If the answer is "yes", then it might be worth it to receive this test. On the other hand, if the answer is "no", which usually is the case, then it's probably best not to get this test.

Chapter Summary

- Hyperthyroidism in the presence of elevated thyroid stimulating immunoglobulins is usually diagnostic of Graves' disease.
- It's important to know that while most people with an autoimmune thyroid condition will have positive thyroid antibodies, it's also possible to have false negative antibodies.
- Although the Radioactive Iodine Uptake test probably won't cause permanent damage to your thyroid gland, it usually won't change the course of treatment, and this is true even if someone has thyroid nodules.
- Women who are pregnant or breastfeeding shouldn't receive the radioactive iodine uptake test.

For access to the book references and resources, visit
savemythyroid.com/hyperbooknotes

CHAPTER 18

5 Reasons To Avoid Radioactive Iodine Treatment

WHEN JIM WAS DIAGNOSED with Graves' disease, two different endocrinologists recommended for him to receive radioactive iodine treatment. Although he had moderate hyperthyroid symptoms, they were being controlled by the antithyroid drugs he was taking. Even before he stumbled upon my website he was opposed to having his thyroid gland obliterated, and so he continued taking PTU to help manage his hyperthyroid symptoms (he initially was prescribed methimazole but had a negative reaction). Like many people who consult with me for the first time, Jim was very skeptical of natural treatment methods. However, he didn't want to take the antithyroid drugs for a prolonged period of time, and he wanted to do everything he could to avoid radioactive iodine.

So he consulted with me, and after discussing his test results he began following my recommendations. He experienced some positive changes in his symptoms, although there wasn't much of a change in his thyroid blood tests after he retested for the first time (after two months had gone by). I told him not to become discouraged, as everyone is different, and it was great that his symptoms had started to improve.

He continued following the recommendations, saw an improvement in his blood test results two months later, and the next time he had retested (a couple of months later) his thyroid panel had normalized, and a few months later his thyroid stimulating immunoglobulins also were normal. While many people in Jim's situation would have followed the advice of their endocrinologist and received the radioactive iodine, Jim realized that radioactive iodine should be the last resort in most cases.

In the United States, radioactive iodine is commonly recommended as the first line of treatment for people with hyperthyroidism. Sometimes this happens even when the person's hyperthyroid symptoms are mild. I have personally consulted with people with mild hyperthyroid symptoms who had their thyroid gland obliterated through radioactive iodine. Many endocrinologists will recommend RAI based on the thyroid blood tests alone. In other words, if someone has a low TSH and/or high thyroid hormone levels, they will recommend radioactive iodine to that patient, regardless of how mild their symptoms might be.

The following represent five reasons why radioactive iodine should usually be the last resort:

Reason #1: Receiving radioactive iodine will most likely make you hypothyroid for the rest of your life. Because radioactive iodine obliterates the thyroid gland, most people will develop hypothyroidism. As a result, most of these people will need to take synthetic or desiccated thyroid hormone for the rest of their life. While many people do fine on thyroid hormone replacement, why damage or destroy your thyroid gland if you don't have to? The thyroid gland is one of the most important parts of the body, and shouldn't be obliterated or removed unless absolutely necessary.

Reason #2: Many people do fine taking antithyroid drugs. When I spoke with an endocrinologist upon being diagnosed with Graves' disease, she was somewhat conservative, and she didn't recommend radioactive iodine to me. Instead she prescribed antithyroid drugs, which I didn't take, but I did respect her for not being too aggressive right off the bat. Even though antithyroid drugs won't cure hyperthyroidism, in my opinion they are definitely a better first option when compared to radioactive iodine.

I realize that side effects are common with antithyroid drugs such as methimazole, PTU, and carbimazole. And if this describes you then you might need to look into other options, such as bugleweed or cholestyramine (I discuss cholestyramine in Chapter 28). But while side effects are common, if you can tolerate antithyroid medication then in most cases it's at the very least a better option than radioactive iodine or thyroid surgery.

Although I can't say that I love antithyroid drugs, there is no denying that they do a good job of managing the symptoms in most people with hyperthyroidism. Some people will go into a state of remission while taking antithyroid drugs, although this usually is temporary since most people don't address the underlying cause of their condition. But many people who won't even consider natural treatment methods have done well taking antithyroid drugs for a prolonged period of time.

In fact, studies show that hyperthyroidism can be controlled with antithyroid drugs with only rare exceptions. Could this be the reason why many endocrinologists who practice outside of the United States recommend antithyroid medication first, and perhaps explain why even some endocrinologists in the United States are strongly opposed to radioactive iodine treatment? Once again, some people don't respond well when taking antithyroid medication, and some people have adverse reactions to this medication and therefore are unable to take it. While I realize that not everyone can tolerate antithyroid medication, to not at least attempt to manage the person's symptoms in this manner before recommending a treatment that damages their thyroid gland is ludicrous.

Reason #3: Radioactive iodine can lead to other serious health issues. While radioactive iodine will usually eliminate the hyperthyroid symptoms, this harsh treatment method doesn't do anything for the actual cause of the condition. This of course is why I recommend a natural treatment approach, as my goal is to always try to get to the underlying cause of the person's condition. And since the thyroid gland isn't the actual cause of the problem in most cases, many people who receive radioactive iodine will develop other health issues in the future.

If becoming permanently hypothyroid isn't enough to discourage you from receiving radioactive iodine, then how about this piece of research: "long-term follow-up studies have revealed an increased cardiovascular mortality in those with a past history of hyperthyroidism treated with RAI".[195]

Another study showed that "Among patients with hyperthyroidism treated with radioiodine, mortality from all causes and mortality due to cardiovascular and cerebrovascular disease and fracture are increased".[196]

These studies were included in the second edition of the book, but upon doing some updated research I came across a journal article which showed that radioactive iodine was associated with an increased risk for mortality from overall cancer, breast cancer, and non-breast solid cancers.[197] I came across another study that looked to quantify the risks of malignancies associated with RAI treatment for children and young adults.[198] The conclusion was that the RAI treatment was associated with increased risks of several solid cancers, particularly more than 20 years after exposure.

The next study I came across is significant for those women who are of childbearing age and are thinking of conceiving in the future. The objective of the study was to assess the impact that RAI may have on fertility in women.[199] This was a smaller study involving 51 women, 40 who were exposed to RAI, and 11 who were only treated with a thyroidectomy. Of the women who received RAI, 40% went through early menopause, while no cases were reported among the controls. The authors concluded that RAI can affect a woman's fertility and shorten her reproductive life.

Reason #4: The quality of life is worse for those who receive radioactive iodine. This isn't me just saying this, as this is according to the research. Although earlier studies show that quality of life is similar among patients treated by antithyroid drugs, radioactive iodine, or thyroid surgery, a more recent study didn't confirm this.[200]

This study involved 1,186 patients with Graves' disease. 347 patients were treated with antithyroid drugs only, 395 patients treated with radioactive iodine, and 233 patients treated with surgery. Quality of life was assessed using two different questionnaires on an average of eight years after the diagnosis of Graves' disease.

Among the three treatment groups, patients who received radioactive iodine treatment had worse thyroid-specific quality of life scores than patients treated with antithyroid drugs or surgery. The radioactive iodine therapy group had worse scores for the following: hyperthyroid symptoms, goiter symptoms, fatigue, anxiety, depression, emotional susceptibility, impaired social life, impaired daily life, and impaired sex life. In addition, the study also showed that those who received radioactive iodine had worse scores in hypothyroid symptoms as well as eye symptoms and appearance than the antithyroid drug group.

It's important to mention that both the patients in the surgery group and the antithyroid drug group were younger than those in the radioactive iodine group: 54 years compared to those of 35 years in the surgery group and 43 for the antithyroid drug group. More patients in the radioactive iodine therapy group had other medical conditions that may affect quality of life. But these factors alone didn't explain the decreased quality of life.

Reason #5: Radioactive iodine might cause or exacerbate thyroid eye disease. Not only do studies show this, but I have also seen people receive radioactive iodine and develop thyroid eye disease or experience an exacerbation of their existing thyroid eye disease condition.

In the former case, the person probably had mild thyroid eye disease without symptoms, and then when they received radioactive iodine, they developed overt eye symptoms. While many endocrinologists won't recommend radioactive iodine treatment for those with active thyroid eye disease, this doesn't mean that radioactive iodine can't cause overt thyroid eye disease in those without eye symptoms. So you want to be very cautious.

How does radioactive iodine cause or exacerbate thyroid eye disease? Apparently, radioactive iodine leads to prolonged worsening of autoimmunity against the TSH receptor. Taking steroids after receiving radioactive iodine might prevent an exacerbation of thyroid eye disease, so this is something to consider if you do choose radioactive iodine. This is especially true for someone who has had Graves' disease for less than five years, as there is an increased risk for reactivation of thyroid eye disease.

Why Can't Endocrinologists Agree Which Treatment Method Is The Best?

What's amazing is that endocrinologists can't even agree with regards to which treatment methods patients should receive. When I was doing my research for this book, I came across various different opinions, and here is an example of the opinions held by four different endocrinologists:[201]

"I treat almost everyone with propylthiouracil (PTU). I avoid 131I (radioactive iodine) in all patients unless there are reasons to the contrary. I have not recommended surgery in 15 years for such patients."

"All my patients are given the option of selecting 131I, surgery, or antithyroid drugs. I advise 131I as the simplest, safest, cheapest, decisive treatment. Ninety percent accept this advice".

"There is no question that time and experience world-wide have shown that 131I is the treatment of choice for thyrotoxicosis"

"We remain conservative with regard to radioiodine in patients of childbearing and child-siring age. Because of the persistence of leukocyte chromosomal breakage for years after radioiodine therapy, we would like to see the F1 generation assurances of the safety of radioiodine".

When Is Radioactive Iodine Really Necessary?

So when is radioactive iodine treatment really necessary to receive? Well, I'd like to say that if I had to choose between radioactive iodine and thyroid surgery I would without question choose the latter option, and so I'm not sure if anyone can conclude that there is a time and place when RAI treatment is truly "necessary". That being said, here are two of the primary situations when radioactive iodine might be considered:

1. **When every other treatment option has failed.** As I already discussed, in most cases, people with hyperthyroidism should choose to take anti-thyroid drugs to manage the symptoms before receiving radioactive iodine. Although these prescription drugs won't cure hyperthyroidism, they usually do a good job of managing the symptoms, might lower the thyroid antibodies, and sometimes will put a person into a state of remission, although most of the time it's temporary. But in most cases this option is definitely better than obliterating your thyroid gland, and ideally you would want to do things to improve your health when taking the antithyroid medication.

Speaking of which, you know that I recommend a natural treatment approach to people with hyperthyroidism, as while not everyone can be helped through natural treatment methods, many people can regain their health. It admittedly is a challenge to take a natural treatment approach, which is a reason why some people choose radioactive iodine. After all, it's much easier to receive radioactive iodine treatment than to take a natural treatment approach. But when you think about how important the thyroid gland is to your health, it is well worth making the "sacrifice" to restore your health.

What approach should someone take if they have a negative reaction to the antithyroid medication? If someone is sensitive to methimazole, then they might do fine taking PTU, and vice versa. On the other hand, some people are sensitive to both types of antithyroid medication. If this is the case then there are a few different options.

First of all, one can consider using natural antithyroid agents such as bugleweed and/or higher doses of L-carnitine to manage the symptoms.

Of course everyone is different, and for some people these natural agents aren't potent enough to lower the thyroid hormones. If this is the case then two other options to consider before resorting to radioactive iodine are 1) cholestyramine and 2) low dose naltrexone (LDN). I talk about both of these in Chapter 28.

2. **Certain Cases Of Thyroid Cancer.** If you have thyroid cancer then you very well might need to receive radioactive iodine or thyroid surgery. That being said, there are natural health experts who focus on cancer, although I can't say that I'm one of them. If I had thyroid cancer I'm honestly not sure what approach I would take, but since most cases of thyroid cancer are slow-growing and aren't fatal I'd like to think that I would at least consider a natural treatment approach (while working with an expert), but it's easy for me to say this when I'm not personally dealing with thyroid cancer.

Getting back to radioactive iodine, just remember that if you choose to receive this treatment, this still doesn't correct the cause of the problem. Whether someone has hyperthyroidism or thyroid cancer, there still were factors which led to the development of these conditions. This is why it's not a bad idea for someone who has already received RAI to work with a natural healthcare professional, as they still have triggers and underlying imbalances that should be addressed.

It's also important to mention that although many people who receive RAI do fine on thyroid hormone replacement, some people still have moderate to severe symptoms. As you know by now, RAI doesn't do anything for the immune system component of Graves' disease, doesn't address compromised adrenal glands, won't improve the health of your gut microbiome, etc. In summary, radioactive iodine won't do anything to remove the triggers and other underlying imbalances which resulted in the thyroid or autoimmune thyroid condition in the first place.

I realize that for some people it can be tough to choose a natural treatment approach when an endocrinologist tells you that RAI is necessary. After all, they're perceived as being a health expert, which is why many with hyperthyroidism end up receiving this procedure. But one shouldn't take obliteration of their thyroid gland lightly. As a result, if a doctor recommends for you to receive radioactive iodine and you're not sure if this is the right decision, consider what I have discussed.

After all, you only have one thyroid gland, and you want to do everything you can to keep it if at all possible. As I mentioned earlier, if I had to choose between radioactive iodine treatment and thyroid surgery I'm pretty sure I would choose a thyroidectomy. Of course I'm hoping that I'll continue to maintain a state of wellness and won't ever need to choose between the two. And I realize that there are also risks associated with thyroid surgery, which is why I would also try everything you can to avoid this as well.

Still Skeptical About the Risks Of Radioactive Iodine? Then Please Read The Following

For those who still are skeptical about the risks of radioactive iodine, keep in mind that those who receive radioactive iodine are instructed to take certain precautions the first few days after receiving this treatment. This includes using separate towels and bed linens, different plates and silverware, etc. They are also advised to sleep in a separate bed from their partner, and to avoid kissing and engaging in sexual intercourse for a few days after receiving radioactive iodine.

Some doctors will advise people who have received radioactive iodine treatment to flush the toilet a few times after using the bathroom in order to dilute the amount of radiation in the urine and feces. In some countries, people who receive radioactive iodine are quarantined for a few days. Remember that this is radiation we're talking about, and so while many people with hyperthyroidism choose to receive this treatment method, any medical doctor who claims that it's completely harmless is either naive or is being dishonest.

Can Someone Benefit From Natural Treatment Methods AFTER Receiving Radioactive Iodine?

Some people who have already received radioactive iodine might wonder whether they would benefit from natural treatment methods. As for whether your thyroid gland can regenerate, it depends on the extent of damage which was done to the thyroid gland, which usually is dependent on the dosage of radioactive iodine that was used. The good news is that just because you received radioactive iodine treatment doesn't mean you can't benefit from a natural treatment approach. This is true even if you have become hypothyroid.

The reason for this is because the body has an amazing ability to heal. While a person who has a thyroid gland that was completely removed through surgery or one that was damaged extensively through RAI very well might need to take thyroid hormone for the rest of their life, partial damage or partial removal of this gland still offers some hope of being able to restore your health through a natural treatment approach.

Many people who have received radioactive iodine become depressed and sometimes even angry when they realize that they might have had a chance to "save" their thyroid gland instead of permanently damaging it through this treatment. But once again, if you received radioactive iodine treatment you still might be able to be helped through natural treatment methods. In fact, the question really isn't whether or not you can benefit from natural treatment methods, but whether or not you can have your thyroid health restored. As for completely restoring your thyroid health, this admittedly is more difficult to accomplish after receiving radioactive iodine, although sometimes it still is possible depending on the amount of damage which was done to the thyroid gland.

For those people who received radioactive iodine and can't have their health restored through a natural treatment approach, they still can usually benefit from natural treatment methods. The reason for this is because radioactive iodine does nothing for the actual cause of the hyperthyroid condition. While it is usually effective in eliminating the hyperthyroid symptoms, just remember that in most cases the thyroid gland isn't the cause of the hyperthyroid disorder, as I have mentioned numerous times already.

So as you know by now, the goal of a natural treatment approach is not just to manage your symptoms, but to get to the underlying cause of the condition. Sometimes natural treatment methods will be able to assist in restoring the thyroid function of the individual who has received radioactive iodine. Other times it's not possible to completely restore a person's thyroid health, but it is still is important to restore the health of other areas of their body which led to the development of their disorder, which will help to prevent future conditions from developing.

Getting Over The Anger Of Receiving Radioactive Iodine

As I briefly mentioned previously, after learning that a natural treatment approach can potentially help with hyperthyroidism, some people who have already received radioactive iodine become upset, and even angry that they received this treatment. If this describes you, I can understand your frustration. The truth is that while radioactive iodine should be considered as a last resort, what you need to understand is that this is how most endocrinologists and other medical doctors are trained to treat such conditions.

While there are some great endocrinologists in practice, most are trained to use drugs and radioactive iodine as their primary treatment methods for hyperthyroid conditions. In fact, if you were to ask your endocrinologist or general medical practitioner about natural treatment methods, chances are they would advise you not to follow through with such a protocol.

As I have already mentioned in this book, even though I'm a natural healthcare practitioner, I honestly was skeptical before I took a natural treatment approach for Graves' disease. And while I'd like to think that my Graves' disease condition has been cured, I'd be thrilled if I continue maintaining my health for many years to come. All I know is that I was feeling great after taking a natural treatment approach, was still feeling great after writing the first and second editions of this book, and now as I put together the third edition of this book almost a decade later I'm feeling better than I ever have before, and of course have no regrets about the choices I have made.

But for those people who have already received radioactive iodine treatment, please don't give up hope. There still is a chance that the function of your thyroid gland can be restored through a natural treatment approach. It admittedly will be more challenging when compared with someone who hasn't received radioactive iodine, but restoring your health is still a possibility. And even if this isn't the case, just remember that what originally caused your hyperthyroid condition to develop probably still exists. Because of this, at the very least you should consider natural treatment methods to "optimize" your health and to prevent other conditions from developing in the future.

Chapter Summary

- The following represent three reasons why radioactive iodine should usually be the last resort: 1) Receiving radioactive iodine will most likely make you hypothyroid for the rest of your life. 2) Some people do fine while taking antithyroid drugs, and 3) radioactive iodine doesn't do anything for the underlying cause of the condition.
- Here are two of the primary situations when radioactive iodine treatment might truly be necessary: 1) When every other treatment option has failed and 2) with certain cases of thyroid cancer
- Just because you received radioactive iodine therapy doesn't mean you can't benefit from natural treatment methods.
- The only way to truly determine whether someone who has received radioactive iodine therapy can be helped through natural treatment methods is to actually give them a try. The good news is that it usually doesn't take too long to see if these treatment methods are helping.

For access to the book references and resources, visit
savemythyroid.com/hyperbooknotes

CHAPTER 19

The Risks Of Playing
The Waiting Game

WHEN BELINDA WAS DIAGNOSED with Graves' disease by her endocrinologist, the doctor was conservative and didn't recommend radioactive iodine. Instead, she told Belinda to take methimazole to manage the hyperthyroid symptoms. Her advice was to take the methimazole for 18 months, and to see if her condition goes into a state of remission. Belinda took the methimazole, and sure enough, her Graves' disease condition went into remission, and after the 18 months had passed she was able to stop taking the antithyroid medication.

Of course the antithyroid drugs didn't do anything for the underlying cause of the condition, so it shouldn't have been a surprise when about eight months later she began experiencing hyperthyroid symptoms again. Belinda went back to her endocrinologist, who put her back on the methimazole, but warned Belinda that she might need to receive radioactive iodine to permanently "fix" the problem.

At the time Belinda was an email subscriber on my website, and after reading some of my articles and watching some of the videos on my website she decided she wanted to work with me. To make a long story short, upon taking a natural treatment approach Belinda's symptoms subsided in about one month, her thyroid markers gradually improved and eventually normalized, and she learned how to maintain her health in order to prevent a relapse from occurring.

Many people with hyperthyroidism who don't receive radioactive iodine will take antithyroid medication. Taking antithyroid drugs definitely is a more conservative option than receiving radioactive iodine. And for many people, antithyroid drugs do a good job of managing their hyperthyroid symptoms. Methimazole and propylthiouracil (PTU) are two of the more popular antithyroid drugs taken by many people with hyperthyroidism.

Taking antithyroid medication can be wise for some people who have hyperthyroidism. After all, hyperthyroid symptoms can at times be severe, and it's risky to deal with a very high pulse rate, severe palpitations, etc. So without question, some people do need to take antithyroid drugs to help manage their symptoms. Of course this assumes they are well tolerated, as side effects are common.

Antithyroid Drugs Are Usually A Temporary Solution

While antithyroid drugs will usually help to manage someone's hyperthyroid symptoms, in my opinion they should only be used on a temporary basis in the majority of cases. Of course for someone who is not looking to take a natural treatment approach, then perhaps taking antithyroid medication is the best long term option, as there are studies that show that it's safe to take low dose methimazole on a long term basis (once again, for those who are able to tolerate it). The problem is that many people take antithyroid drugs and pray their condition will go into a state of remission.

While some people do go into a state of remission when taking antithyroid drugs, many people don't. Plus, many people who do go into a state of remission will eventually relapse in the future. So what may happen is that someone who is taking antithyroid drugs for one or two years may go into a state of remission, but after a few months or years the hyperthyroidism is likely to return, and when this happens they will most likely end up receiving radioactive iodine or thyroid surgery.

Of course the reason for the relapse is because the cause of the condition was never addressed. Once again, the antithyroid medication may do a good job of managing the symptoms, but they won't do anything for the underlying cause of the hyperthyroid condition. So the person who takes these drugs and goes into a state of remission but then doesn't address the actual cause will never have their health restored.

It's Risky To Aim For A Remission Through Taking Drugs

In Chapter 6 I spoke about the difference between remission and cure, and I discussed how someone with hyperthyroidism might suffer a relapse, even if they restore their health through natural treatment methods. Because of this, you might wonder what's the difference between suffering a relapse when taking antithyroid drugs when compared to taking a natural treatment approach? After all, it's easy to take medication, but it can be challenging to take a natural treatment approach. Plus, if someone takes a natural treatment approach, neglects their health, and suffers a relapse, they probably will need to go through the process again.

However, one has to consider a few things. First of all, even though it sounds like I'm encouraging the use of antithyroid drugs in this chapter, the truth is that side effects are common with methimazole, PTU, etc. Remember that I personally didn't take antithyroid medication, but I realize some people need to do so, and in most cases this is a better option than radioactive iodine or thyroid surgery. The second thing a person needs to consider is that antithyroid drugs don't do anything for the actual cause of the condition. So for example, even if someone with a hyperthyroid condition who has adrenal imbalances and a compromised immune system responds well while taking antithyroid drugs, this isn't doing anything for adrenal imbalances or a compromised immune system.

So not only is someone who goes into remission very likely to relapse, but this person I just described has a good chance of developing other autoimmune conditions, as I explained in a previous chapter. So in this example it would be important for them to address both the adrenal glands and the immune system component. Similarly, if they had digestive issues or a high toxic burden, taking antithyroid drugs wouldn't do anything to help with these.

Side Effects Of Antithyroid Medication and Beta Blockers

Although it's completely fine for people to take antithyroid medication and/or beta blockers while taking a natural treatment approach, at the same time I think it's a good idea to be familiar with some of the common side effects. While not everyone has a negative reaction to antithyroid medication, a lot of people experience minor side effects, while some experience moderate to severe side effects.

Methimazole: Some of the more common side effects include itching, hives, hair loss, weight gain, swelling, joint or muscle aches, heartburn, and headaches. Elevated liver enzymes are also common. Less common side effects include a decreased white blood cell count. Studies show that methimazole is usually more effective in managing the hyperthyroid symptoms and in the induction of euthyroidism when compared to PTU.[202] This is one of the main reasons why methimazole is commonly recommended over PTU, but it's not the only reason, which I'll discuss next.

Propylthiouracil (PTU): The side effects of this antithyroid medication are very similar to those of methimazole. However, some people who experience side effects with methimazole do fine when taking PTU, and vice versa. And so if you took one type of antithyroid medication and didn't do well, it might be worth trying a different type. One potential concern with PTU is that it can be harsher on the liver, and there is some evidence that it can cause liver failure,[203] although this is extremely rare, and I'll say here that over the years I've had a good number of patients take PTU without a problem.

It's also important to mention that both methimazole and PTU have been shown to have negative effects on the gut microbiome. The research shows that these antithyroid drugs caused changes in the gut microbiota structure, and the drug-induced side effects were associated with LPS production and intestinal barrier destruction.[204, 205] LPS stands for lipopolysaccharides, which are large molecules found in gram-negative bacteria that can cause a leaky gut.[206, 207]

Beta Blockers (i.e. Propranolol, Atenolol): Although beta blockers can do a great job of helping to manage the cardiac symptoms associated with hyperthyroidism, symptoms are common. Some common symptoms include nausea, vomiting, and stomach cramps. But in some cases taking beta blockers can cause headaches, dizziness, and in rare cases even hallucinations. I haven't had any of my patients experience hallucinations, but I have had a few experience dizziness due to taking beta blockers, along with some of the other symptoms I listed.

Just a reminder that in Chapter 12 I discussed how some beta blockers can inhibit mitochondrial CoQ10 enzymes. And so if you're taking a beta blocker then you might want to consider supplementing with CoQ10.

If You're Looking For A Quick Cure...

Without question it is more challenging to address the underlying cause of your hyperthyroid condition than to take prescription drugs. I commonly mention how people who aren't willing to take responsibility for their health shouldn't bother consulting with a natural healthcare professional. I wish it were an easy process, but the truth is that it usually takes many years for hyperthyroid conditions such as Graves' disease and toxic multinodular goiter to develop, so it's ridiculous to expect a quick and easy cure.

Antithyroid drugs can provide a quick solution to manage the symptoms while at the same time trying to address the underlying cause of your condition. But by no means should these drugs be looked at as being a cure. Some people don't mind taking antithyroid drugs, which is fine. However, if you're looking to address the actual cause of your condition and would like to attempt to restore your health, which I'm guessing you're interested in since you're reading this book, then even if you choose to take antithyroid medication you should strongly consider addressing the underlying cause of your hyperthyroid condition.

Chapter Summary

- While antithyroid drugs can help manage someone's hyperthyroid symptoms, in my opinion they should only be taken on a temporary basis in most cases.
- While some people do go into a state of remission when taking antithyroid drugs, many people don't. Plus, many people who do go into a state of remission will eventually relapse in the future since they didn't do anything to address the underlying cause.
- Not only is someone who goes into remission while taking antithyroid drugs very likely to relapse, but there is a risk of developing other autoimmune conditions in the future
- The truth is that it takes many years for hyperthyroid conditions such as Graves' Disease and toxic multinodular goiter to develop, so it's unreasonable to expect a quick cure.

For access to the book references and resources, visit
savemythyroid.com/hyperbooknotes

CHAPTER 20

Combining Natural Treatment Methods With Conventional Treatment Methods

TERRI WAS INTERESTED IN taking a natural treatment approach, but she was concerned about stopping her thyroid medication. By reading some of the articles on my website she realized that she could address the underlying cause of her hyperthyroid condition while taking the antithyroid drugs. When I consulted with her for the first time I told her that it would be fine for her to take the antithyroid medication while taking a natural treatment approach, and that only she can make the decision to wean off the antithyroid drugs.

And that's exactly what happened, as she felt better upon following my recommendations and her thyroid blood tests improved. Since the TSH was on the high side she advised her endocrinologist that she was going to reduce the dose of antithyroid medication on her own, and hopefully get to the point where she didn't need the medication. Her endocrinologist wasn't happy to hear this, and told her that making diet and lifestyle changes wouldn't be of any help. Well, Terri successfully weaned herself off of the drugs, and because she continues to maintain her health she continues to feel great to this day.

Some people are hesitant to give natural treatment methods a try because they are concerned about stopping the prescription medication they are taking for their hyperthyroid condition. I will never tell any of my patients to stop taking antithyroid drugs. I might tell someone my story about when I was diagnosed with Graves' disease and how I personally decided not to take any antithyroid medication.

But I will never tell anyone to stop taking their medication, as this is only a decision they can make on their own. In fact, there are times when I think it's a good idea for people with hyperthyroid conditions to take the antithyroid drugs on a temporary basis to help manage their symptoms. But ultimately it's up to the patient to decide what they want to do.

So for those people who want to give natural treatment methods a try but at the same time want to continue taking their current medication, there is no rule which says they can't continue taking antithyroid drugs and/or beta blockers and still take a natural treatment approach. Of course there might be some contraindications regarding certain supplements and herbs which normally would be recommended if you weren't taking any prescription drugs, but a competent natural healthcare professional should be able to advise the patient what supplements and/or herbs they can and cannot take while taking thyroid medication.

When I was diagnosed with Graves' disease, I had the option of taking the antithyroid drugs and the beta blocker, and then I still could have taken a natural treatment approach. If I took this approach then as my health improved eventually I would have weaned off the medication. This definitely was an option I considered, but I decided to not take the antithyroid drugs or beta blocker, as I just took a natural treatment approach and used bugleweed and motherwort to manage the hyperthyroid symptoms, which turned out to be a great decision on my part.

What Is The Best Option For You?

As far as what you should do, once again, this is a decision that only you can make. I will say that people with hyperthyroidism are more at risk when they don't manage their symptoms when compared with someone who has hypothyroidism, and therefore they might want to consider taking antithyroid drugs if their symptoms are severe. So for someone who has a very high pulse rate and severe heart palpitations, it might be a good idea to take the antithyroid drugs and/or a beta blocker, and at the same time take a natural treatment approach. This again is just an option, as I'm not trying to recommend that anyone who has been diagnosed with a hyperthyroid condition should make this choice.

As I briefly mentioned earlier, for some people with hyperthyroidism, it's a good idea for them to continue taking their antithyroid medication while addressing the underlying cause of their condition. Even though fatalities with hyperthyroidism and Graves' disease are rare, there definitely are risks of uncontrolled hyperthyroidism, and anyone who has a high pulse rate or any other cardiac symptoms needs to manage these symptoms. Plus, atrial fibrillation is common in hyperthyroidism,[208, 209] and this is another reason why it's important to manage the hyperthyroid symptoms.

If you're currently not taking antithyroid drugs then one question you may have is "how high should my resting pulse rate be before I decide to take medication?" There is no specific answer to this, as all I can say is that people with moderate to severe symptoms definitely need to manage their symptoms. Plus you need to keep in mind that it's not just about the cardiovascular risks, as elevated thyroid hormones can also have a negative effect on bone density.[210, 211]

This is important to understand, as every now and then I'll work with someone who has elevated thyroid hormones, yet doesn't have an elevated resting heart rate. Because of this they may think that there aren't any concerns, but even if you aren't experiencing any overt symptoms, hyperthyroidism can decrease bone density, and in some cases can even lead to osteoporosis. I also came across a study that showed that TSH receptor antibodies associated with Graves' disease may also have a negative effect on bone density.[212]

Are Bugleweed & Motherwort Good Substitutes For Antithyroid Drugs?

In the chapter where I talked about nutritional supplements and herbs (Chapter 12), I spoke about the herbs bugleweed and motherwort, and how they can help a great deal with the symptoms in many people with hyperthyroidism and Graves' disease. And there are many people who decide not to take the antithyroid drugs or beta blockers, but instead take one or both of these herbs. However, while these herbs are great, sometimes they aren't potent enough to manage a person's hyperthyroid symptoms, especially if they are severe. This is also true with emergency situations such as thyroid storm, as someone with this condition definitely shouldn't rely on herbs to manage their symptoms.

But even when the symptoms aren't considered to be life threatening, which is the case with most people who have hyperthyroidism, you do need to be careful about just taking these or any other herbs as substitutes for antithyroid drugs. I'm of course not suggesting that these herbs aren't effective, as I used them to manage my hyperthyroid symptoms when I was diagnosed with Graves' disease, and many of my patients use them to manage their hyperthyroid symptoms as well. All I'm trying to say is that they aren't always adequate substitutes for antithyroid drugs and beta blockers, as for some people looking to take a natural treatment approach, the medication will do a better job of managing the person's symptoms until the natural treatment protocol begins to take effect.

This is just something you need to keep in mind, as while both bugleweed and motherwort work well for many people with hyperthyroidism, I've also had patients who took both bugleweed and motherwort and who didn't notice much of a difference in their symptoms after taking these herbs for some time. This doesn't mean the herbs aren't effective, but for some people they aren't potent enough to effectively manage the symptoms.

Taking Antithyroid Medication For A Prolonged Period Of Time

Some people choose to take the antithyroid medication for the amount of time their medical doctor recommended and at the same time take a natural treatment approach. In other words, they don't wean off of the antithyroid drugs a few months into the natural treatment protocol, but they instead take the medication for as long as they were told to by their doctor. For example, if they were told to take methimazole or PTU for 18 months, then some will take it for the full 18 months, and at the same time take a natural treatment approach.

While most of the people I consult with prefer not to take the antithyroid drugs for a prolonged period of time, I have no problem working with someone who chooses this option. What usually happens is that the thyroid hormone levels will start decreasing in those people who are taking antithyroid medication and at the same time taking a natural treatment approach. As a result, the endocrinologist will usually reduce the dosage of medication due to these changes.

However, some endocrinologists will still recommend for the patient to continue taking a very small dose of methimazole (i.e. 5 mg/day) even when the thyroid hormone levels and TSH are within normal limits.[213] I'll talk more about this option in Chapter 28, as while the goal of this book is to help people restore their health so that they don't need to rely on taking antithyroid medication on a long term basis, everything comes down to risks vs. benefits. In other words, if someone is struggling to restore their health, and if the natural symptom management options (i.e. bugleweed, L-carnitine) aren't effective, then in my opinion, taking lower doses of methimazole (if tolerated) is a better option than receiving radioactive iodine or thyroid surgery.

It's Best To Consult With Your Endocrinologist or General Medical Practitioner

Whenever someone with hyperthyroidism consults with me and is taking antithyroid medication, I always give them the different options they have. Some will choose to continue taking the medication, while others will want to stop taking it and substitute the medication with herbs such as bugleweed and motherwort. For those who choose the latter option, I always refer the patient back to their primary care physician just so it is known that it wasn't I who made the decision for the patient to stop taking their medication, but instead it was a decision made between the patient and their medical doctor. Some patients will choose not to speak with their medical doctor but will just stop taking the medication on their own.

That being said, many medical doctors, including most endocrinologists, won't approve of any patient taking a natural treatment approach. As a result, I let the patient know that while they should consult with their medical doctor about the different options they have, there is a good chance their doctor won't approve of them following such a protocol. And a big reason for this is because they don't have a good knowledge about natural treatment methods, and most don't want to open their minds to these methods. This of course doesn't describe every medical doctor, as fortunately there are some medical doctors that practice functional medicine who understand how safe and effective natural treatment methods can be.

In any case, it is the person with hyperthyroidism who needs to make this decision as to whether they should stop taking the prescription medication, or continue taking drugs while taking a natural treatment approach. Even if they speak with an endocrinologist or another type of medical doctor who is open to natural treatment methods, it ultimately is the patient who will need to make the decision. The goal of the natural healthcare professional is to give the patient all of the information they need in order to make an informed decision, and not to make the actual decision for the patient.

How Will You Know When It's Time To Wean Off Your Medication?

As I mentioned before, I never tell someone to wean off or stop taking their medication. But as someone takes a natural treatment approach and begins to restore their health, the thyroid hormone levels eventually should decrease, and the TSH should of course increase. The only way to know if this is happening is to monitor the TSH and thyroid hormone levels regularly.

As the thyroid hormone levels decrease most endocrinologists won't have a choice but to reduce the dosage of medication in order to prevent you from becoming hypothyroid. Keep in mind that it's common for the TSH to take a little longer to increase. In other words, the thyroid hormone levels frequently will normalize while the TSH remains low.

To summarize this chapter, for anyone with hyperthyroidism who is currently taking antithyroid drugs, or is considering taking them, it is fine to combine both conventional and natural treatment methods. Taking the prescription drugs usually won't prevent someone from restoring their health, and in fact could be important if the hyperthyroid symptoms are severe. While many people want to try to avoid taking any type of medication if at all possible, at the same time you need to be smart about this, as you need to weigh the benefits and risks in this situation.

Chapter Summary

- For those people who want to give natural treatment methods a try but at the same time want to continue taking their current medication, there is no rule which says they can't continue taking antithyroid drugs and still take a natural treatment approach.
- For someone who has a high resting pulse rate and heart palpitations, it might be a good idea to take the antithyroid drugs and/or a beta blocker, and then follow the natural treatment protocol while weaning themselves off of the drugs under the supervision of their endocrinologist.
- Although the herbs bugleweed and motherwort can do an excellent job of managing a person's symptoms, they shouldn't be viewed as a substitute for antithyroid drugs for people with severe hyperthyroid symptoms.
- It is the person with the hyperthyroid condition who needs to make this decision as to whether they should stop taking drugs, or continue taking drugs while following a natural treatment protocol.

For access to the book references and resources, visit
savemythyroid.com/hyperbooknotes

CHAPTER 21

Can Thyroid Nodules Be Treated Naturally?

BARBARA'S THYROID ULTRASOUND revealed two thyroid nodules, one which was 0.7 cm in size, and the other was 1.6 cm in size. Her endocrinologist wanted to do a biopsy for the larger nodule, but Barbara preferred not to get a biopsy. Upon consulting with me we did some initial testing, and a few of her blood test markers suggested that she had insulin resistance, and she also did dried urine testing, which demonstrated high 4-OH metabolites, which essentially means that she had problems with estrogen metabolism.

Although I can never guarantee that someone's thyroid nodules will shrink over time, over the years I have seen this happen with many patients by addressing the underlying imbalances. And so I of course gave recommendations to help address Barbara's insulin resistance and estrogen metabolism problems. After six months of following the recommendations she got another ultrasound done, and while both thyroid nodules were still present, they had decreased in size, as the first one decreased from 0.7 cm to 0.4 cm, and the larger one decreased from 1.6 cm to 1.1 cm.

Many people with hyperthyroidism have thyroid nodules, which are abnormal growths of thyroid tissue. In most cases, thyroid nodules aren't anything to be concerned about, but sometimes they can cause problems which need to be addressed. Many times endocrinologists will recommend for a person with thyroid nodules to take extreme actions, even when they aren't causing any issues. So the goal of this chapter is to discuss why thyroid nodules develop, as well as some of the different treatment options available, including natural treatment options, surgery, radiofrequency ablation, and castor oil packs.

I want to start off by letting you know that it is very common for people to have thyroid nodules. One journal article mentioned that while 4 to 7% of the population has palpable thyroid nodules, ultrasonography reveals that up to 67% of the population has them.[214] Another study mentioned that up to 35% of the population have thyroid nodules show up on an ultrasound.[215] Even if we go with the lower number, 35% is quite high, as this means that roughly one third of the population has thyroid nodules. The incidence of thyroid nodules increases as we age, and the prevalence is higher in women,[215] although they are more likely to be malignant in men, especially those over 70 years of age.[216]

Two Common Causes of Thyroid Nodules

Problems with estrogen metabolism. According to the research, estrogen is a potent growth factor both for benign and malignant thyroid cells.[217, 218] Estrogen is also a factor with uterine fibroids, and one study involving 1144 participants looked at the relationship between thyroid nodules and uterine fibroids.[219] The authors concluded that uterine fibroids in women were definitely associated with the presence of thyroid nodules, and that estrogen might play a pivotal role in the occurrence of both of these.

As a result, if you have one or more thyroid nodules, doing things to support estrogen metabolism is a good idea. One of the best ways to accomplish this is by eating plenty of cruciferous vegetables, as these help to support estrogen metabolism due to the compounds Indole-3-Carbinol and 3,3'-diindolylmethane (DIM).[220, 221] Another option is to take DIM in supplement form, although you wouldn't want to do this if you have low estrogen levels, as it can also further decrease them.

It's also important to mention that there is a relationship between estrogen and the gut microbiome.[222, 223] In other words, having imbalances in the gut microbiome (dysbiosis) can cause problems with estrogen metabolism. And the reason for this is because the gut microbiota regulates estrogens, and if someone has dysbiosis this can impair the excretion of estrogen from the body, which in turn can be a factor in the development of thyroid nodules.

Insulin Resistance. Insulin is a hormone that is produced by the beta cells of the pancreas. As the name implies, insulin resistance is when the cells are no longer sensitive to insulin. So this is a high insulin state, which is why this is associated with pre-diabetes and type 2 diabetes. Although some doctors rely on a fasting glucose test to determine if someone has insulin resistance, other testing is recommended to make a diagnosis, including a fasting insulin and a hemoglobin A1C. Elevated triglycerides on a lipid panel (in a fasting state) can also be a sign of insulin resistance.

As for how insulin resistance develops, eating a diet consisting of high amounts of refined carbohydrates and sugars is without question a factor. Consuming high amounts of fructose can especially be problematic, as this can lead to an increase in fat deposition in the liver and skeletal muscle, thus increasing the risk of insulin resistance and type 2 diabetes.[224]

Inflammation plays a role in insulin resistance, and there are many different causes of inflammation. Since the mitochondria play a role in glucose homeostasis, mitochondrial dysfunction can also be a potential cause. There is even evidence that intestinal dysbiosis (an imbalance of the gut flora) can be a factor in insulin resistance,[225] which is yet another reason to do everything you can to improve the health of your gut microbiome.

The following are situations when someone who has thyroid nodules should consider using medical intervention:

1. **If the thyroid nodule is malignant.** If the thyroid nodule is malignant, then this is an obvious situation which requires medical intervention. Some sources show that less than 1% of all thyroid nodules are malignant,[226] although one study stated that the reported prevalence of malignancy in thyroid nodules evaluated by biopsy ranges from 4% to 6.5%, and is largely independent of the nodule size.[227] If the nodule is cold on the radioactive iodine uptake scan then there is a greater chance of it being malignant, which is the argument some endocrinologists will make to have you do this test. Just keep in mind that the majority of cold nodules are also benign as well.

   When it comes to determining if someone has a malignancy, numerous studies have shown that a fine needle aspiration of the thyroid gland is the most reliable and cost-effective method of distinguishing benign from malignant thyroid nodules.[228, 229] However, fine needle aspiration is far from perfect, and more recently genetic testing has been used to determine whether someone has a malignant thyroid nodule. [230] If the thyroid nodule is found to be malignant, then surgery of the thyroid nodule and/or the thyroid gland itself will most likely be recommended.

2. **When there is a physical obstruction caused by the thyroid nodule.** If the thyroid nodule is very large and is causing an obstruction, leading to difficulty with swallowing and/or breathing, then this is another obvious example of where medical intervention is required. Once again, in these situations, surgical removal of the thyroid nodule or the actual thyroid gland is usually recommended. However, radiofrequency ablation might be another option to consider, and I'll discuss this shortly.

3. **If the thyroid nodule is causing excess secretion of thyroid hormone.** If hyperthyroidism results due to one or more thyroid nodules, then this is yet another reason why medical intervention might be required. While radioactive iodine treatment or surgery is frequently recommended under these circumstances, another option is to take antithyroid drugs to control the symptoms, and then at the same time take a natural thyroid treatment approach in an attempt to shrink the thyroid nodule. Even though this approach isn't always effective, in my opinion it's definitely worth giving it a try in order to possibly prevent thyroid surgery. Another option is radiofrequency ablation, which once again, I'll discuss soon.

4. **When there is any other pain or discomfort due to the presence of the thyroid nodule.** If the thyroid nodule is causing any type of pain or physical discomfort, then medical intervention will most likely be required. This is yet another scenario where surgical removal of the thyroid nodule may be recommended.

When Is Surgery For Thyroid Nodules Really Necessary?

For many of these problems involving thyroid nodules that I just mentioned, surgery of the thyroid gland itself will be recommended. While surgery will most likely resolve the problems previously listed, there are potential risks involved with thyroid surgery. One risk is that the person is most likely to become hypothyroid, which of course is a certainty if the entire thyroid gland is removed. But even with a partial thyroidectomy there still is a decent chance of the person becoming hypothyroid. If this happens then they will be advised to take synthetic or desiccated thyroid hormone for the rest of their life.

Of course in some cases, complete removal of the thyroid gland might be necessary. But if at all possible, removal of the thyroid nodule alone would be a much better option. This not only will take care of the problem, but will also leave much of the thyroid gland intact, which is the ideal scenario. Even though there still is the chance of the person becoming hypothyroid in this situation, there is also the chance they won't develop hypothyroidism, and therefore won't need to take thyroid hormone for the rest of their life.

Unfortunately they usually won't perform surgery of a single thyroid nodule, but earlier I mentioned radiofrequency ablation, which is another option to consider. And unlike radioactive iodine or thyroid surgery, radiofrequency ablation preserves the health of the thyroid gland. I promise that I will be discussing this treatment option soon!

Another potential risk of receiving surgery of the thyroid gland is that it can cause damage to some of the surrounding structures, including the parathyroid glands and the laryngeal nerve. These problems are more common than you would think, and is yet another reason why thyroid surgery should be avoided if at all possible. Once again, I realize this isn't always possible, but if your endocrinologist tells you that surgery of the thyroid gland is necessary, you probably will want to receive a second opinion.

And if you do decide to get thyroid surgery I would make sure to choose a surgeon who has a lot of experience with thyroidectomies. You want to try to choose a surgeon that performs at least 20 thyroidectomies a year. 50 or more would be even better. This is from the research I have done. If you choose someone who does 50 a year, and they have been in practice for 10 years, that's 500 thyroid surgeries.

One study showed there was an 87% chance of complications in surgeons who have done only one operation a year, 68% for 2-5 cases, 42% for 6-10 cases, 22% for 11-15 cases, 10% for 16-20 cases, and only 3% for 21-25 cases.[231] Those who did more thyroid surgeries had a similar rate of complications. So as I mentioned earlier, ideally you want to choose a surgeon that does at least 20 thyroid surgeries per year, and despite what the research says, in my opinion more would be better.

Just as is the case with radioactive iodine, many endocrinologists can't agree with one another with regards to the approach to take with thyroid nodules. To no surprise, studies show that surgeons are more in favor of surgery of thyroid nodules when compared to non-surgeons. Another study showed that "only malignant or large symptomatic nodules require surgical excision".[232] The same study showed that "fine-needle aspiration, biopsy, guided by ultrasonography when possible, results in substantial reduction of unnecessary surgery". In other words, some surgeries can be prevented simply by doing thorough testing.

However, as I mentioned earlier in this chapter, a biopsy won't always conclude if a thyroid nodule is malignant or benign. I also mentioned that there is genetic testing available which supposedly is more accurate, but also is very expensive. Perhaps the cost of this testing will go down in the future.

When is a Thyroid Biopsy Necessary?

Although I mentioned that a biopsy can result in a significant reduction of unnecessary thyroid surgeries, this doesn't mean that everyone who has one or more thyroid nodules should consider getting a biopsy. In fact, even some people who have one or more larger thyroid nodules might not need to get a biopsy.

For those who are considering having a biopsy done, I would read the article "Too Many Unnecessary Thyroid Biopsies Performed". This is based on a report in JAMA internal Medicine (218) which involved 8806 patients, and three ultrasound nodule characteristics—microcalcifications, size greater than 2 cm, and an entirely solid composition—were the only findings associated with the risk of thyroid cancer.

Based on these findings the authors of the study suggested that rather than performing a biopsy of all thyroid nodules larger than 5mm, one should instead require two abnormal nodule characteristics to determine if someone should require a biopsy. They mention how this would reduce unnecessary biopsies by 90% while maintaining a low risk of cancer.

To summarize, according to the study I just mentioned, if someone has a thyroid nodule and is concerned about it being malignant, it probably would be best to hold off on getting a biopsy unless if they had at least two of the following three characteristics:

1) Microcalcifications of the thyroid nodule
2) A nodule size greater than 2 cm
3) An entirely solid composition

What About Toxic Multinodular Goiter?

Some people have a condition known as toxic multinodular goiter, also known as Plummer's disease. This involves an enlarged thyroid gland, and also consists of numerous nodules which result in the excess production of thyroid hormone. Although this condition usually affects women who are older than 60 years of age, I have seen younger people with this condition as well. Either way, the person will have hyperthyroid symptoms, but unlike Graves' disease, the thyroid antibodies are usually negative, and as a result most people with this condition also don't have any eye involvement.

Just as is the case with Graves' disease, with toxic multinodular goiter, most endocrinologists will recommend antithyroid medication, RAI, or thyroid surgery.[234] One study suggested that there can be a high incidence of complications if the procedure is not carried out by surgeons with experience in endocrine surgery.[235] Although I've had some success helping people with multinodular goiter, it does seem to be more challenging to restore someone's health with this condition.

But the primary goal will be the same, which is to try to find the underlying cause of the condition, address the cause, and help the person achieve overall optimal health. This is also accomplished by having the person eat well, manage their stress, improving estrogen metabolism, recommending nutritional supplements, etc. I have dedicated a separate chapter (Chapter 25) where I further discuss multinodular goiter.

Can Taking a Natural Treatment Approach Help Prevent Surgery?

Is it possible to shrink the thyroid nodule by taking a natural treatment approach, and thus avoid surgery? In most cases the answer to this question is "yes", although there are situations that require immediate intervention.

And if natural treatment methods were successful in shrinking the thyroid nodule, this still takes time to accomplish. Someone with a serious obstruction probably wouldn't be able to wait for the effects of the natural treatment methods to take place. So while taking a natural treatment approach might help to shrink the thyroid nodule over time, in some cases immediate intervention is necessary.

On the other hand, if you have one or more thyroid nodules that aren't "suspicious" or causing an obstruction, then it very well might be worth giving a natural treatment approach a try. Taking this approach can potentially help preserve your thyroid gland and allow you to avoid taking thyroid hormone for the rest of your life. So I do recommend natural treatment methods in cases where the thyroid nodule isn't malignant, and isn't causing an obstruction or any severe symptoms.

Of course some people want a guarantee that their thyroid nodules will shrink by taking a natural treatment approach. Obviously no doctor can make such a guarantee, as it's not as if there is some "magic" supplement or herb which will shrink thyroid nodules. But by taking a natural treatment approach and balancing the person's thyroid hormone levels, along with correcting any estrogen metabolism problems, as well as insulin resistance (if it's present), many times the thyroid nodules will decrease in size.

And let's not forget that taking a natural treatment approach won't just help benefit your thyroid health, but your overall health as well. So even if you take a natural treatment approach but it doesn't shrink any thyroid nodules you may have, it's not as if following the protocol was a complete waste, as it will benefit your health in many other ways.

What You Need To Know About Radiofrequency Ablation

Radiofrequency ablation (RFA) is a treatment that is performed under ultrasound guidance, and it involves thermally ablating the thyroid nodules, while preserving the health of the thyroid gland. So if someone has one or more larger nodules and surgery is indicated, while I would consider taking a natural treatment approach, RFA is another option to consider. And this treatment can be used for autonomously functioning thyroid nodules.[236] Some of the potential side effects include a transient voice change, hyperthyroidism, hematoma, skin burn, edema, coughing, and nausea/vomiting.[237]

If you want to learn more about RFA then I'd recommend checking out episode #70 of my podcast, where I interviewed Dr. Angela Mazza. You can check out the episode by visiting savemythyroid.com/70. Dr. Mazza is board certified in internal medicine, diabetes, endocrinology and metabolism, and performs RFA. There are other practitioners as well who perform this procedure.

Can Iodine Shrink Thyroid Nodules?

There is some evidence which shows that iodine can shrink thyroid nodules. Dr. Guy Abraham has done a lot of research when it comes to iodine, and he has come to the following conclusion: "Thyroid nodules respond positively to iodine/iodide supplementation. Serial ultrasounds usually show a decrease in the size of the thyroid cysts and nodules and eventual resolution of the lesions."[238] Another study concluded that nodules are frequently associated with Graves' disease in iodine deficient areas[239], although the study didn't discuss whether iodine supplementation can help to shrink thyroid nodules.

Although I'm very cautious when it comes to iodine supplementation in those with hyperthyroidism, my experience is that iodine can be helpful in some cases of thyroid nodules. Quite frankly, not all of my patients who have one or more thyroid nodules receive a follow-up ultrasound to show whether or not the thyroid nodules have decreased in size after iodine supplementation. In any case, I think that iodine can potentially help some people with thyroid nodules, but this doesn't mean that I recommend for everyone with thyroid nodules to supplement with iodine. As I explained in Chapter 13, I'm not "anti-iodine", but I'm very cautious when it comes to recommending iodine supplements in those with thyroid and autoimmune thyroid conditions.

Prior to supplementing with iodine I would look into the two potential causes of thyroid nodules I mentioned at the beginning of this chapter: problems with estrogen metabolism and insulin resistance. And if you do decide to look into iodine supplementation I would consider doing a urinary test for iodine, and I would also highly recommend working with a practitioner who has experience with recommending iodine supplementation.

Can Castor Oil Packs Shrink Thyroid Nodules?

To no surprise, there is no research which proves that castor oil packs can help shrink thyroid nodules. This doesn't mean much, as just because no research studies have been conducted doesn't mean that certain natural treatment methods aren't effective. One problem is that sometimes thyroid nodules will shrink on their own, and so if one uses castor oil packs and they help to shrink the thyroid nodules, there really is no way to tell if this would have occurred without the castor oil packs. Similarly, some people who take a natural treatment approach will have their thyroid nodules shrink, but perhaps in some cases this would have happened even if they didn't do anything naturally.

When I wrote the first and second editions of the book I didn't have much experience using castor oil packs on my patients, and I mentioned that "using castor oil packs have a low risk, but probably come with a low reward." And I still think this is true, but I should mention that in 2023 I interviewed Carrie Vitt on my podcast, who spoke about using castor oil packs, and the benefits they have when it comes to thyroid nodules. To listen to this episode visit savemythyroid.com/87.

In summary, if you have hyperthyroidism, along with one or more thyroid nodules, and have been told by your endocrinologist that surgery to remove the nodule or thyroid gland itself is necessary, it's a good idea to obtain a second opinion. And if you aren't experiencing severe symptoms, then you very well might want to consider speaking with a competent natural healthcare practitioner to see if natural treatment methods might be able to help you. While there are no guarantees that you can shrink your thyroid nodule naturally, it is a much more conservative approach than receiving surgery, radioactive iodine, or any other extreme medical procedures. And of course if the natural treatment approach is successful in shrinking the thyroid nodule it will most likely help you to avoid thyroid surgery or RAI, and if it's not successful then radiofrequency ablation is another option to consider..

Chapter Summary

- Many times endocrinologists will recommend that a person with thyroid nodules take extreme actions, even when they aren't causing any issues.
- The following are situations when someone with a hyperthyroid condition who has thyroid nodules should consider choosing medical intervention: 1) if the thyroid nodule is malignant, 2) when there is a physical obstruction caused by the thyroid nodule, 3) if the thyroid nodule is causing excess secretion of thyroid hormone, 4) when there is any other pain or discomfort due to the presence of the thyroid nodule
- In some cases, partial or complete removal of the thyroid gland might be necessary, but there are other options to consider, such as radiofrequency ablation..
- Radiofrequency ablation (RFA) is a treatment that involves thermally ablating the thyroid nodules, while preserving the health of the thyroid gland
- Even if you take a natural treatment approach but it doesn't shrink any thyroid nodules you have, it's not as if following the protocol was a complete waste, as it will benefit your health in many other ways.

For access to the book references and resources, visit
savemythyroid.com/hyperbooknotes

CHAPTER 22

Overcoming Thyroid
Eye Disease

TIFFANY CAME TO SEE me for her Graves' disease condition, and she actually found me through a thyroid eye disease workshop I was hosting at the time. During the workshop I admitted that in some cases conventional treatment is necessary for thyroid eye disease, especially for more severe cases. Thankfully Tiffany's case wasn't severe, but she was experiencing eye pressure, and her eye bulging was noticeable to close family members and friends.

Prior to working with me she took low dose naltrexone (discussed in Chapter 28), but she didn't notice any difference after being on it for a few months. She considered taking Tepezza if her health insurance covered it, and she might have ended up taking it if she didn't come across my workshop. By attending my workshop Tiffany learned that thyroid eye disease can be reversed naturally in many cases, depending on the severity.

While working on finding and removing her triggers (after doing some testing) she decided to take the supplements in my TED Bundle to help with the symptoms and reduce some of the inflammation. It took a few months before her eyes started improving, but she started noticing the pressure decreasing, and eventually the eye bulging improved.

Thyroid Eye Disease (TED), also known as Graves' ophthalmopathy, is an inflammatory eye condition which affects many people with Graves' disease. It involves the same antibodies associated with Graves' disease (thyroid stimulating immunoglobulins), as these antibodies can also attack the tissues of the eyes. Studies show that Graves' ophthalmopathy is clinically relevant in approximately 50% of patients with Graves' disease, with severe forms affecting 3 to 5% of patients.[240] The good news is that this condition will self-resolve in many people, but it still can cause long-lasting problems, most commonly exophthalmos (bulging eyes).

Although this condition usually self-resolves, sometimes conventional medical treatment is necessary to help manage the symptoms. For example, corticosteroids are used in some cases to help with the inflammation. And in some cases more extreme treatment methods are used, such as radiation, immunosuppressant drugs, and sometimes even surgery. And in 2020 a new treatment option was introduced called Teprotumumab, sold under the brand name Tepezza, which I'll discuss later in this chapter.

Natural Treatment Methods To The Rescue?

Can natural treatment methods reverse thyroid eye disease (TED), or prevent it from developing in someone who currently isn't stricken with this condition? Let's first answer the second question. If someone has Graves' disease and is taking a natural treatment approach, and if this is successful in restoring their health then in most cases the person won't develop TED. And even if this doesn't completely restore their health, since the natural treatment approach will help to greatly improve their immune system health, there still is a good chance it will prevent the occurrence of TED. This once again is based on the experience I have had with my patients.

On the other hand, for someone who already has TED, natural treatment methods still can usually help. This doesn't mean that natural treatment methods will always help with TED, and it is definitely more challenging with severe cases. For example, if someone has a severe case of exophthalmos, taking a natural treatment approach may not completely reverse this.

Does this mean that someone with severe TED shouldn't take a natural treatment approach? Not necessarily, as while there are cases where those with TED can't fully restore their health, in many cases taking a natural treatment approach can still help greatly, or at the very least manage the symptoms without the person having to worry about the side effects which are common with conventional medical treatment. So while there are no guarantees, it definitely is worth a try in my opinion.

The Risks Of Receiving Radioactive Iodine Treatment With Thyroid Eye Disease

I mentioned the potential risks of radioactive iodine in Chapter 18, including how it can cause TED. Some studies show that radioactive iodine therapy is associated with an increased risk of thyroid eye disease,[241, 242] although this doesn't happen in all patients who receive RAI. By now you know that I'm not a big fan of radioactive iodine, and of course this is true even when people don't have TED. While some people choose to receive radioactive iodine, it usually should be a last resort, after everything else has been tried. So whether or not you have TED, in my biased opinion I would highly recommend that you at least consider giving natural treatment methods a try first, unless if it's a medical emergency which requires you to receive conventional medical treatment.

For those people who do receive radioactive iodine treatment and experience an increase in their TED symptoms, in most cases corticosteroids will be recommended. If you have TED and have received RAI, and are now experiencing a worsening of your symptoms, you might wonder at this point whether or not natural treatment methods would be effective. Even with people who have received radioactive iodine treatment, natural treatment methods can potentially help with TED.

While it is less likely that someone who has received radioactive iodine treatment can have their thyroid health restored, it still is possible to suppress the autoimmune component of the condition. And since it is the immune system which is causing the problems with the eyes, addressing the autoimmune component is still important in those who have received radioactive iodine treatment.

Can Diet and Lifestyle Help with Thyroid Eye Disease?

You probably already know the answer to this question, as eating a healthy anti-inflammatory diet can benefit many people with TED. And since chronic stress and lack of sleep can contribute to the inflammatory process, working on stress management and getting sufficient sleep can also play an important role. That being said, the impact that diet and lifestyle has on TED will vary from person to person. In some people diet and lifestyle alone will lead to a dramatic improvement in one's eye symptoms, but others may not notice much of a difference.

While nobody likes to give up their favorite foods, I do think it's still important to eat a healthy diet for the reasons discussed in Chapter 11. While you might want to consider following an autoimmune Paleo (AIP) diet, at the very least I would take a break from eating common allergens such as gluten, dairy, corn, and soy, along with avoiding the nightshades. Even if you don't notice symptomatic improvement, continuing to eat these foods can have a negative effect on your gut microbiome, which in turn can make it more challenging to reverse your TED condition.

What Supplements Or Herbs Can You Take To Help With Thyroid Eye Disease?

As I've already discussed in this chapter, Graves' ophthalmopathy is caused by the thyroid stimulating immunoglobulins attacking the tissues of the eyes. And the autoimmune component is responsible for the thyroid antibodies. And so in order to help with TED, one needs to suppress the autoimmune component and do things to help with the inflammation.

While a lot can be accomplished through diet and lifestyle, there are a number of different nutritional supplements and herbs which can potentially help with thyroid eye disease. I've already discussed some of them in Chapter 12, as some of the same supplements that can benefit Graves' disease can also benefit TED, which makes sense since 1) they are both autoimmune conditions and 2) most people with TED have Graves' disease.

Selenium. I can probably write an entire chapter on the benefits of selenium, and since I already spoke about this mineral in Chapter 12 I'll make it short and sweet, as numerous studies show that selenium can benefit those with thyroid autoimmunity, as well as thyroid eye disease.[243, 244, 245] The dose will depend on the person, although it's not uncommon for healthcare professionals to recommend 200 mcg to 400 mcg of selenium per day to their patients. However, selenium toxicity is a concern, and so I would be cautious about taking high doses of selenium for a prolonged period of time.

Vitamin D. I can also write an entire chapter on vitamin D, and I also discussed this in Chapter 12. While vitamin D is important for bone health, the research shows that a vitamin D deficiency is an independent risk factor for thyroid eye disease.[246] Although you want to get as much vitamin D as you can from the sun, supplementation with vitamin D3 is frequently necessary. As for dosing, it really depends on the levels, which is why I recommend a 25-OH vitamin D test to all of my patients. And as I mentioned in Chapter 12, if I recommend vitamin D3 I also would take vitamin K2, as it helps to guide the calcium into the bone.

Omega 3 Fatty acids. I also mentioned this in Chapter 12, although I'll add that you might want to go on the higher side with the dosage of EPA and DHA. I mentioned how I usually recommend between 1,000 to 2,000 mg of eicosapentaenoic acid (EPA) and 500 to 1,000 mg of docosahexaenoic acid (DHA), and so I recommend for my patients with TED to take closer to 2,000 mg of EPA and 1,000 mg of DHA.

Alpha lipoic acid (ALA). this is a well known antioxidant, and it has been shown to regenerate endogenous antioxidants, including vitamin C, vitamin E, and glutathione.[247] I came across a study that showed that alpha lipoic acid can inhibit oxidative stress-induced adipogenesis in orbital fibroblasts in people with Graves' ophthalmopathy.[248] A fibroblast is a type of cell that is responsible for making the extracellular matrix and collagen, and studies show that it may play a role in TED.[249] As for dosing, if I recommend ALA to my TED patients I typically will advise them to take 100 to 200 mg per day.

Berberine. For many years I would recommend berberine for its antimicrobial and blood sugar balancing properties. And I still think it can greatly benefit people with blood sugar imbalances such as insulin resistance and type 2 diabetes, and also can help with certain infections. But there is also evidence that it has inhibitory effects on tissue remodeling in orbital fibroblasts.[250] In addition, evidence shows that it has modulatory effects on the gut microbiota,[251] and by now you know that a healthy gut is necessary for a healthy immune system.

In Chapter 15 I discussed how berberine is the most abundant alkaloid in the herb Goldenseal. I also mentioned that it can be effective in eradicating certain infections, which can in turn be a trigger of Graves' disease and TED. Some are concerned that berberine might have negative effects on some of the commensal bacteria in the gastrointestinal tract, but the more recent research shows that it has beneficial effects on the gut microbiome.

Quercetin. Quercetin is a member of the flavonoid family contained in vegetables and fruits, and while I commonly recommend it to those with a histamine intolerance, it also has anti-inflammatory, antioxidant, and anti-viral activity.[252] And a few different studies show that it can benefit those with thyroid eye disease.[253, 254]

Resveratrol. I briefly mentioned resveratrol in Chapter 12, and I'll add that the research shows that resveratrol can reduce ROS levels and inhibit adipogenesis in the orbital fibroblasts in thyroid eye disease patients.[255]

Curcumin. I also mentioned turmeric/curcumin in Chapter 12, and the research shows that curcumin inhibits proinflammatory cytokine production, ROS synthesis, and adipogenesis in orbital fibroblasts of thyroid eye disease patients.[256]

It's important to mention that some of these studies are in vitro (test tube) studies, and in vitro studies don't always translate to real life situations. That being said, over the years I've had a lot of TED patients take these supplements, and some of them are included in my Thyroid Eye Disease bundle, which you can check out by visiting TEDbundle.com.

Should Tepezza Be Considered?

The way Tepezza works is by binding to the Insulin-like growth factor 1 receptor (IGF-1R), which causes degradation of the antibody-receptor complex. Elevated levels of the IGF-1 receptor have been found in orbital fibroblasts as well as B and T cells from patients with Graves' disease.[257] Apparently IGF-1R forms a complex with the TSH receptor, and inhibiting this complex can greatly help people with thyroid eye disease.

Tepezza has been shown in trials to decrease proptosis, double vision, and other symptoms associated with moderate to severe cases of thyroid eye disease. Unlike other non-surgical options for thyroid eye disease (i.e. corticosteroids), teprotumumab can stop the progression of thyroid eye disease.

Tepezza has to be administered through intravenous infusions, which of course is a major inconvenience. The good news is that it's only given once every 3 weeks for a total of 8 infusions. The dose depends on the patient's weight, and the starting dose used in the studies is 10 mg/kg, followed by 20 mg/kg.

Side Effects and Contraindications

Just like most other conventional medical treatments, side effects are common with Tepezza. These are some of the potential side effects of teprotumumab:

- Muscle cramps
- Spasms
- Nausea
- Hair loss
- Diarrhea
- Fatigue

- High Blood pressure
- Hearing problems
- Taste changes
- Headache
- Dry skin

It's also worth mentioning that as of writing this book, there is a lawsuit related to Tepezza, as in some cases it has caused permanent hearing loss or tinnitus. I've had a few patients take Tepezza, and one of them experienced hearing loss, although it was temporary. But besides the potential side effects, Tepezza is also very expensive if you don't have health insurance, and perhaps most importantly, it isn't doing anything to address the cause of the TED condition.

Can Low Dose Naltrexone Help With TED?

I discuss low dose naltrexone (LDN) in Chapter 28, as it's a prescription medication that can help to modulate the immune system. As a result, a lot of practitioners recommend it for different types of autoimmune conditions. Once again, I'll talk more about LDN in Chapter 28, but I'll say here that in some cases it can be helpful, but it doesn't always work, and it's also not doing anything to address the cause of the autoimmune component.

A Summary Of The Different Treatment Options You Have With Thyroid Eye Disease

Treatment Option #1: Conventional Medical Treatment. As I mentioned before, there are numerous medical treatment approaches depending on your condition. Many people with this condition are prescribed steroids to help with the inflammation. Others with severe TED might receive more aggressive treatment procedures, including surgery. I wouldn't consider Tepezza to be a "conventional" medical treatment for TED since it is a fairly new treatment, but it definitely isn't a natural treatment option, and so I'll still mention it under this category.

I'm not going to sit here and criticize these medical treatments, as there is a time and place for both corticosteroids and surgery. On the other hand, just like any other type of medical treatment, you need to be aware of potential side effects. One study came to the conclusion that there is an urgent need for improved treatment modalities in Graves' ophthalmopathy.[258] So if you do choose the medical treatment option, just keep in mind that this usually is just a temporary solution, although this might be fine since many times this condition will self resolve anyway.

Treatment Option #2: Natural Treatment Options. I'm obviously biased towards using a natural treatment approach, as my goal is always to try to get to the root cause of the problem. Once again, I do think symptom management is important, and because of this, sometimes it is necessary to take prescription drugs. However, in my opinion this should be temporary if at all possible, as if one chooses a natural treatment approach and at the same time takes medication to control their symptoms, then I see nothing wrong with this. On the other hand, for those people who simply take the advice of their medical doctor without wanting to try to restore their health, I'd be lying if I told you that this doesn't frustrate me.

I realize that many people are skeptical when it comes to both the safety and effectiveness of natural treatment methods. I just wonder why they aren't just as concerned about the potential short-term and long-term side effects of the conventional medical treatment methods. When taking a natural treatment approach, in most cases the worst case scenario involves the person not responding to the treatment. With regards to receiving medical treatment, there are a lot of potential risks involved, some of which I have described in this book.

I already discussed the risks of radioactive iodine in Chapter 18, we all know the potential risks that come with any type of surgery, and I mentioned that with Tepezza there is the potential for permanent hearing loss and/or tinnitus. And we even can't take treatment with corticosteroids lightly. Once again, there is a time and place for conventional medical treatment, but my point is that there is usually very little risk in treating mild to moderate cases of TED conditions naturally under the guidance of a competent natural healthcare practitioner, but there can be substantial risks with taking the medical route.

But what about severe cases of Graves' ophthalmopathy? Well, in this case I think natural treatment methods are still worth considering, and I have helped some people with severe cases of Graves' ophthalmopathy, although I'll admit that it's more challenging. If someone has severe eye bulging and/or optic never compression then I definitely would consider medical intervention, and this is especially true in the latter case. I'll add that if someone with a severe case of TED chooses to take a natural treatment approach I do think it's important to also work with a competent ophthalmologist.

Graves' ophthalmopathy is caused by the same thyroid antibodies which attack the TSH receptors.[259] And as you now know, in order to restore someone's health who has Graves' disease, one needs to detect and remove the triggers, suppress the autoimmune component, and control the inflammation. Doing this will usually help with TED as well. In fact, this is the reason why TED will frequently become worse after RAI, as while this treatment will obliterate the thyroid gland, it won't do anything for the autoimmune response, and therefore the thyroid antibodies will continue to attack the tissues of the eyes.

But why isn't this the case with thyroid surgery? In other words, why doesn't thyroid surgery make TED worse? The reason why a complete thyroidectomy typically won't worsen TED is because it removes the entire thyroid gland, whereas with radioactive iodine there usually is still some thyroid tissue left. And as long as there is some thyroid tissue left the immune system will continue to produce TSH receptor antibodies, which can attack the tissues of the eyes.

Treatment Option #3: Combining Conventional & Natural Treatment Methods. Some people want to try to restore their health, but at the same time want to take medication to help manage their symptoms until the natural treatment methods "kick in". As I mentioned earlier, when dealing with a condition such as Graves' disease, not only am I supportive of this approach, but in many cases I would actually recommend it. My concern is not so much the progression of thyroid eye disease, but rather that the symptoms of hyperthyroidism itself can become dangerous, specifically the increased heart rate.

That being said, when it comes specifically to combining conventional treatments for TED with natural treatment options, there are situations where it can be more challenging to restore someone's health. For example, if someone is taking corticosteroids on a long-term basis while following a natural treatment approach, it might be challenging to heal the gut while taking the medication. However, the same can be true with antithyroid medication, as I discussed in Chapter 19 how methimazole and PTU can have a negative effect on the gut microbiome. But I will say that I've had many people take antithyroid medication and yet still be successful in healing their gut.

Can Tepezza be combined with a natural treatment approach? As of writing this book I've only had a few patients on Tepezza, but I will say that they do seem to respond to the natural treatments. Of course when it comes to the changes in their eyes this probably has a lot to do with the Tepezza, but as you know, the Tepezza isn't going to do anything to find and remove triggers, correct underlying imbalances, etc. And while I mentioned some of the immediate side effects of Tepezza earlier, since it's only been out for a few years we still don't know what the potential long-term side effects of Tepezza might be.

Treatment Option #4: No Treatment. Since many cases of TED will self resolve without any intervention, this is yet another option you have. Many people will choose to receive no treatment, especially if their symptoms are mild. If this is the case, you might decide not to choose either medical or natural treatment methods, and hope that the condition goes away on its own and doesn't become any worse. The only concern with this approach is that a mild case of TED can sometimes turn into a moderate or severe case over time, and so you shouldn't be surprised that even in mild cases of TED I would recommend to do things to improve your immune system health.

In summary, thyroid eye disease doesn't affect everyone with Graves' disease, and when it does affect someone, the symptoms are frequently mild and warrant minimal or no treatment. However, in cases where the symptoms are moderate or severe, medical treatment might be able to help manage the symptoms, but you might want to consider a natural treatment approach to get to the underlying cause of this condition. This of course not only will help with the symptoms, but even if you can't completely restore your health, natural treatment methods still can prevent the condition from progressing in many people.

If you want more information on TED I would definitely check out my podcast (Save My Thyroid), and you might want to specifically check out an interview I did with Dr. Rani Banik (savemythyroid.com/26), who is a board-certified ophthalmologist and fellowship-trained neuro-ophthalmologist with additional training in Functional Medicine. I also have created a free "Overcoming TED" guide that you can get by visiting

OvercomingTEDGuide.com. I also should mention that Elaine Moore has a great book on TED entitled "Thyroid Eye Disease: Understanding Graves' Ophthalmopathy".

Chapter Summary

- Thyroid Eye Disease, also known as Graves' ophthalmopathy, involves the same antibodies which attack the thyroid gland, as these antibodies can also attack the tissues of the eyes.
- Although this condition usually self-resolves, sometimes conventional medical treatment is necessary to help manage the symptoms.
- If someone has Graves' Disease and is taking a natural treatment approach, if this is successful in restoring their health back to normal then in most cases it will prevent thyroid eye disease from developing.
- For someone who already has thyroid eye disease, natural treatment methods can still usually help.

For access to the book references and resources, visit
savemythyroid.com/hyperbooknotes

CHAPTER 23

Natural Treatment Methods During Pregnancy & Lactation

FOR THOSE WOMEN with hyperthyroidism who are either pregnant or breastfeeding, there are numerous risks associated with the different hyperthyroid treatment options typically recommended by most endocrinologists. What I plan on doing in this chapter is discussing the risks of these conventional treatment methods, and then I'll talk about natural treatment options for pregnant and lactating women. This way you can use this information in order to make an informed decision as to which treatment you would like to receive.

The Conventional Hyperthyroid Treatment Options:

The most common treatment recommended by endocrinologists and other types of medical doctors for pregnant and lactating women with hyperthyroidism is antithyroid drugs. Methimazole and Propylthiouracil (PTU) are two of the most common drugs prescribed, and they can usually do a pretty good job in managing the symptoms of hyperthyroidism. However, there are potential risks to the baby when taking antithyroid drugs during pregnancy. But the risk of untreated hyperthyroidism is usually greater than taking the antithyroid drugs, which is why most endocrinologists usually recommend the latter option.

PTU is usually recommended during the first trimester, as there is an increased risk of congenital malformation when taking methimazole during the first trimester.[260] Methimazole can lead to fetal anomalies such as aplasia cutis, esophageal atresia, and choanal atresia. PTU crosses the placenta to a lesser extent than methimazole, and leads to less cases of fetal hypothyroidism.[261] However, if the patient is intolerant or sensitive to PTU then methimazole may be used.

For those women with hyperthyroidism who are pregnant or breastfeeding who don't respond well to antithyroid drugs, the next step usually would be for them to receive thyroid surgery. This procedure is rarely performed on pregnant and lactating women, and is usually reserved for those women with severe symptoms who don't respond well to antithyroid drugs. Since thyroid surgery comes with many risks during pregnancy, most medical doctors will try to avoid this procedure if at all possible.

Radioactive Iodine Treatment IS NOT Recommended For Pregnant Or Lactating Women

Radioactive iodine has the potential to obliterate the thyroid gland of the fetus, and as a result, it is not recommended by endocrinologists to women who are pregnant. This should give you a good idea as to how harsh of a treatment method this is, as you want to be cautious with any treatment that has the word "radioactive" in it. So as I've mentioned already in this book, even in people who aren't pregnant or lactating, radioactive iodine shouldn't be the first treatment option, yet many doctors do in fact recommend this to their "non-pregnant" patients as the primary treatment option.

Natural Treatment Options

You probably won't be surprised that I recommend for pregnant women with hyperthyroidism to take a natural treatment approach. This doesn't mean that there isn't a time and place for antithyroid medication, and I'll discuss later in this chapter that there are limitations when it comes to taking natural agents for symptom management, including bugleweed, motherwort, and higher doses of L-carnitine. So from a symptom management perspective it can be challenging to manage the symptoms of hyperthyroidism naturally during pregnancy.

Based on what I just said, you might be wondering if a natural treatment approach is safe for pregnant and lactating women. It depends on what your expectations are, as if you expect to lower your thyroid hormones naturally then you might be disappointed for the reasons I just mentioned. On the other hand, I'm hoping that by now you understand that there is a reason why you developed hyperthyroidism, and that you will incorporate most of the strategies discussed during this book to help restore your health.

Getting back to antithyroid medication, I realize that many pregnant or lactating women with hyperthyroidism won't want to take antithyroid medication...especially those reading this book. If you have subclinical hyperthyroidism (low TSH and normal thyroid hormones) then you might be able to avoid the medication, but if you have elevated thyroid hormones you need to keep in mind that everything comes down to risks vs. benefits. If my wife had hyperthyroidism and was pregnant I'm sure I would prefer for her not to take antithyroid drugs, but I also wouldn't want her to have uncontrolled hyperthyroidism, which in turn would put both her health and the baby's health at risk.

Based on what I just said, many pregnant women with hyperthyroidism will take antithyroid medication while incorporating a natural treatment approach. Many who are breastfeeding will also take the medication, although there will be some women who put their health at risk because they realize that their baby will be exposed to the medication through the breast milk. Once again, I realize that for some women, choosing to take or not to take the antithyroid medication isn't an easy decision, but you really do need to weigh the risks vs. benefits.

Which Nutritional Supplements Are Safe For Pregnant Women?

If you visit your local health food store and look at the supplements and herbs on the shelves, many of them will contain wording which suggests women who are pregnant or lactating need to be cautious when consuming such products. What you need to understand is that many of the nutritional supplements and herbal remedies which have warnings aimed towards pregnant and lactating women aren't necessarily unsafe. With regards to nutrients (vitamins, minerals, etc.), there usually is minimal risk when it comes to giving them to a pregnant woman.

In fact, it is essential for pregnant women to take high quality prenatal vitamins. And since many pregnant women don't eat enough whole, healthy foods, taking some additional nutritional supplements is also a good idea (i.e. omega-3 supplement, probiotics). That being said, there are some minerals where a toxicity is a concern, such as selenium and iron.

Some women are also cautious about taking the fat soluble vitamins (vitamins A, E, D, K) during pregnancy. Without question you do want to be careful about overdosing, although in most cases pregnant women will need to take very high doses to cause any harm to the baby. For example, birth defects due to vitamin A toxicity has been associated with intakes as low as 25,000 IU per day.[262] I never recommend very high doses of vitamin A to my pregnant patients, and so as long as you don't take massive doses of vitamins and minerals there is minimal risk for a toxicity to occur.

Can Herbs Be Harmful During Pregnancy and Lactation?

It's a different story with herbs. While some herbs are safe for pregnant women to take, others can be harmful. To no surprise, no clinical research studies have been done to evaluate the side effects of herbs on pregnant and lactating women. This shouldn't be surprising as I know I wouldn't have wanted my wife to participate in such a study when she was pregnant or while she was breastfeeding our children. But this doesn't mean that all herbs are risky for pregnant women to take.

So there are some herbs I would be cautious about giving during pregnancy and lactation, while others which under no circumstances would I give. For example, let's take a look at the "cautions" for the herb Echinacea as listed on the product packaging of a company I sometimes recommend:

"Not to be used during pregnancy and lactation unless otherwise directed by a qualified health care professional."

Now let's take a look at the wording for bugleweed, which as described in Chapter 12, is an herb I frequently recommend for people with hyperthyroidism (and one that I personally took when I was dealing with Graves' disease):

"Contraindicated in pregnancy and lactation. Contraindicated in hypothyroidism and enlargement of the thyroid without functional disorder".

While both of these herbs issue warnings to pregnant and lactating women, you can see the difference between the two warnings. Echinacea warns that it shouldn't be used during pregnancy UNLESS otherwise directed by a qualified healthcare professional. This means they are essentially putting this verbiage down to protect themselves from litigation, but in some cases Echinacea can be taken by pregnant or lactating women while under the guidance of a competent healthcare professional. On the other hand, bugleweed is clearly contraindicated in pregnancy and lactation, and therefore should not be taken by a pregnant woman under any set of circumstances.

I'm not suggesting for pregnant and lactating women to take Echinacea, as I'm just giving an example. Two other immune system herbs which are supposed to be compatible with breastfeeding include bupleurum and rehmannia (which also helps greatly with the adrenals). For the adrenals, the herb ashwagandha is usually safe to take during pregnancy and lactation, although just a reminder that it's part of the nightshade family.

Some sources suggest the herb licorice shouldn't be taken during pregnancy, while other sources claim that it's fine to take. One study did show that maternal licorice consumption can have a negative impact on the cognitive performance of children.[263] Apparently glycyrrhizin, which is a component of licorice, may impair the placenta, allowing stress hormones to cross from the mother to the baby. Overall I'm very conservative about giving herbs during pregnancy, especially during the first trimester.

I frequently mention in this book, as well as the articles and posts on my website, how people with hyperthyroidism shouldn't self-treat their condition, and this obviously is even more important for pregnant women who have hyperthyroidism. And for those who think nutritional supplements and herbs are completely safe because they are "natural", hopefully I've convinced you that this isn't true, and that there are some risks with taking certain herbs. This isn't only true with regards to pregnant women, but with anyone, and is especially true when people mix herbs, or combine certain herbs with medication they are taking. This is yet another good reason to consult with a competent natural healthcare practitioner.

Can Motherwort Be Taken During Pregnancy and Lactation?

When I went through my training for my herbal certification, my instructor was Kerry Bone, an herbalist who has written numerous textbooks on herbal medicine. Obviously I learned about a lot of different herbs, including bugleweed and motherwort, and I also learned about which herbs were safe during pregnancy and lactation, and which herbs were contraindicated.

For bugleweed, this is what was documented in my required reading: "Pregnancy classification C: Has caused or is associated with a substantial risk of causing harmful effects on the fetus or neonate without causing malformations". It was also labeled as "Lactation classification SD: Strongly discouraged in breastfeeding".

As for motherwort, the following was documented: "Pregnancy classification B3: No increase in frequency of malformation or other harmful effects on the fetus from limited use in women. Evidence of increased fetal damage in animal studies, although the relevance to humans is unknown". It was also labeled as "Lactation classification C: Compatible with breastfeeding".

So bugleweed is essentially contraindicated during pregnancy and strongly discouraged in breastfeeding, while motherwort is probably best to be avoided during pregnancy, but seems to be okay when breastfeeding. After reading this you might wonder if you can manage your symptoms by taking motherwort alone if you're breastfeeding, and the answer would be "yes", although keep in mind that motherwort doesn't have antithyroid properties, and so if you have elevated thyroid hormones, taking motherwort by itself might not be sufficient.

It's worth mentioning that Kerry Bone didn't discuss lemon balm during the training I received. And L-carnitine isn't an herb, and so of course this wasn't covered. But there is nothing in the literature about the safety of higher doses of L-carnitine taking during pregnancy and lactation, which is why I would be cautious about taking it. And while taking a smaller dose (i.e. 500 to 1,000 mg/day) might be okay, it might not be sufficient to manage the hyperthyroidism.

Can Thyroid Antibodies Cause Harm To The Fetus?

When working with pregnant women who have Graves' disease, I've been asked by some of them if the thyroid antibodies can affect the health of the fetus. TSH receptor antibodies do cross the placenta, and can induce neonatal thyrotoxicosis.[264] Frequently the pregnancy itself will suppress the autoimmune component of a condition such as Graves' disease, although this might not happen until later on in the pregnancy. However, I've dealt with some patients whose thyroid antibodies continued to stay high throughout the pregnancy.

Can Eating Goitrogenic Vegetables Help Lower Thyroid Hormones?

I already discussed this in Chapter 11, but I'm bringing it up again here because I mentioned how in the past I recommended raw goitrogenic vegetables (i.e. broccoli, kale) to some of my pregnant women with hyperthyroidism. Goitrogens can interfere with thyroid hormone production, and so I was hoping that this would serve as a natural way of managing the symptoms of pregnant and lactating women with hyperthyroidism. But unfortunately this wasn't effective, and so while I do encourage pregnant women to eat cruciferous vegetables, I can't say that I've seen that eating them raw have any significant impact when it comes to reducing thyroid hormones.

Subclinical Hyperthyroidism and Pregnancy

Subclinical hyperthyroidism is characterized by a low TSH with normal thyroid hormone levels. In most cases, antithyroid medication won't be recommended to pregnant and lactating women with this condition. There aren't too many studies which discuss the relationship between subclinical hyperthyroidism and pregnancy/lactation. However, one study looked to evaluate the pregnancy outcomes in women with this condition, and concluded that subclinical hyperthyroidism is not associated with adverse pregnancy outcomes, and identification of subclinical hyperthyroidism and treatment during pregnancy is unwarranted.[265]

Taking a Natural Treatment Approach BEFORE Pregnancy

The ideal situation would be to begin taking a natural treatment approach before becoming pregnant. If you are already pregnant or breastfeeding then you can still of course benefit from taking a natural treatment approach. But if you have hyperthyroidism and you're not currently pregnant or breastfeeding, but are thinking about becoming pregnant in the near future, then taking a natural treatment approach not only can potentially restore your health, but it will also create a very healthy environment for the baby.

Other than being cautious about taking certain herbs, a pregnant woman can follow most of the other advice given in this book. Of course just like anyone else looking to restore their health, it will be essential for them to make certain changes in their lifestyle, as just taking nutritional supplements and herbs alone won't reverse someone's hyperthyroid condition. So anyone who is pregnant will want to eat well, obtain quality sleep, do a good job of managing their stress, minimize their exposure to environmental toxins, etc. Of course this should be the case for any pregnant woman, and not just someone who has hyperthyroidism.

In summary, being pregnant or breastfeeding shouldn't prevent someone from taking a natural treatment approach, although there might be some modifications as to which supplements and/or herbs they can take. This might affect the recovery process to some extent, but overall taking a natural treatment approach can still greatly benefit the health of both the mother and baby.

Chapter Summary

- For those women with hyperthyroidism who are either pregnant or breastfeeding, there are numerous risks associated with the different hyperthyroid treatment options recommended by most endocrinologists.
- Because a natural treatment approach can potentially restore someone's health, many pregnant and lactating women with hyperthyroidism choose natural treatment methods.
- Many of the nutritional supplements and herbal remedies which have warnings aimed towards pregnant and lactating women aren't necessarily unsafe, as you need to read the warnings carefully.
- If you have hyperthyroidism and you're not currently pregnant or breastfeeding, but are thinking about becoming pregnant, then taking a natural treatment approach not only can potentially restore your health, but it will create a very healthy environment for the baby.

For access to the book references and resources, visit
savemythyroid.com/hyperbooknotes

CHAPTER 24

Can a Natural Treatment Approach Help With a Thyroid Storm?

A SMALL PERCENTAGE of people with hyperthyroidism develop a severe condition known as thyroid storm. Even though this condition doesn't affect too many people with hyperthyroidism, those who are affected by a thyroid storm need to get this addressed immediately. This condition is an emergency situation, and conventional medical treatment is highly recommended.

With that being said, can a natural treatment approach play any role in helping people with thyroid storm? Before I answer this, let's look at some of the common symptoms of this condition. People who have a thyroid storm may experience an increased heart rate exceeding 200 beats per minute. They may also experience heart palpitations, an increase in blood pressure, as well as chest pain and/or a shortness of breath. So it's easy to understand why this is considered to be an emergency situation, and why anyone who experiences a thyroid storm needs to see a medical doctor immediately.

But why does someone develop a thyroid storm? Although anyone with a hyperthyroid condition can develop a thyroid storm, there is usually a precipitating event,[266] such as an infection or another stressor on the body. In addition, someone who doesn't manage their hyperthyroid symptoms will also be at increased risk of developing thyroid storm.

Managing The Symptoms Of a Thyroid Storm

Due to the severity of the symptoms, usually a combination of different prescription drugs is used to manage the symptoms of a thyroid storm. Some of the common drugs recommended to people with this condition include beta blockers, antithyroid drugs, and can also include a blockade iodine drug. Sometimes an infection can be causing or contributing to thyroid storm, and when this is the case this obviously needs to be addressed, although this can be challenging if a virus is the underlying cause.

As for taking a natural treatment approach, you might wonder whether someone with thyroid storm can take certain nutritional supplements and/or herbs to help manage their symptoms. Even though there are some herbs which can help manage the symptoms of hyperthyroidism, such as bugleweed and motherwort, these herbs will usually take some time to "kick in". And when someone has a pulse exceeding 200 beats per minute or has difficulty breathing, they obviously don't have time to wait for natural treatment methods to take effect.

Higher doses of L-carnitine (2,000 to 4,000 mg/day) have antithyroid properties, and a few studies have shown that it can help with a thyroid storm.[267, 268] One of these involved taking L-carnitine with low doses of methimazole.[268] Although it's great that these studies demonstrate the effectiveness of L-carnitine, I wouldn't rely on L-carnitine alone to manage a thyroid storm.

Can Natural Treatment Methods Trigger Thyroid Storm?

In the past I've had some people ask whether taking a natural treatment approach can lead to someone developing a thyroid storm. I haven't experienced anyone developing thyroid storm due to taking a specific nutritional supplement or herb. As I mentioned earlier, a thyroid storm happens due to a precipitating event, or when one isn't able to effectively manage the hyperthyroid symptoms.

So for example, if someone with hyperthyroidism refuses to take anti-thyroid medication and/or beta blockers, and if the natural agents are ineffective in lowering the thyroid hormones, then it is more likely for this person to develop a thyroid storm. This doesn't mean it's impossible to develop a thyroid storm if you're taking antithyroid medication and/or beta blockers. But it's less likely to happen.

It's also possible to develop thyroid storm if someone takes large doses of iodine. Even in this case it's rare, but of course I would refer to Chapter 13 to read about my thoughts on iodine supplementation in those with hyperthyroidism.

Preventing a Thyroid Storm From Occurring

Although someone shouldn't use natural treatment methods to manage the symptoms of a thyroid storm, if someone does develop a thyroid storm, after conventional medical treatment methods are used to control the symptoms, then one can use natural treatment methods to attempt to restore the person's health, and prevent another thyroid storm from reoccurring. So at this point one can take antithyroid agents such as bugleweed and/or L-carnitine to manage the hyperthyroid symptoms, and other nutritional supplements and/or herbs to address other imbalances.

Of course just taking supplements and herbs alone won't restore your health, and as a result it's always wise to consult with a competent natural healthcare practitioner, rather than self-treat your own condition (as I've already stated numerous times in this book). After all, while many people don't want to take antithyroid drugs continuously, you also shouldn't need to take bugleweed, L-carnitine, or any other natural agent for symptom management on a permanent basis. The goal should be to get to the underlying cause of the condition if at all possible, and restore your health so you won't need to depend on any medication or herbs.

So for anyone with a thyroid storm who has a "natural mindset", while I can understand the temptation to address it naturally, it's important to seek immediate medical attention. Then once you have the symptoms under control you can take a natural treatment approach to get to the underlying cause of the hyperthyroid condition, and this in turn should help prevent having a future incidence of this condition.

Chapter Summary

- A small percentage of people with hyperthyroidism develop a severe condition known as a thyroid storm, which is an emergency situation, and immediate conventional medical treatment is required.
- Due to the severity of the symptoms, usually a combination of different prescription drugs is used to manage the symptoms of a thyroid storm.
- Even though there are some herbs which can help manage the symptoms of hyperthyroidism, these herbs will take some time to "kick in". And when someone has a pulse exceeding 200 beats per minute or has difficulty breathing, they obviously don't have time to wait for natural treatment methods to take effect.
- After conventional medical treatment methods are used to control a thyroid storm, then one can use natural treatment methods to attempt to restore the person's health, and prevent another thyroid storm from reoccurring.

For access to the book references and resources, visit
savemythyroid.com/hyperbooknotes

a goiter and/or nodules is common with both hypothyroidism and hyperthyroidism. An elevated TSH is usually indicative of low or depressed thyroid hormone levels, which can be caused by an iodine deficiency, goitrogenic substances (which can inhibit thyroid function), and/or other factors that can disrupt thyroid hormone production. Many people with an elevated TSH have Hashimoto's thyroiditis, which like Graves' disease, is an autoimmune thyroid condition. In fact, this is the most common reason why someone has an elevated TSH.

Smoking, stress, certain drugs. Although one of the studies listed "smoking, stress, and certain drugs" as potential causes, there isn't a lot of evidence in the research showing that cigarette smoking causes a multinodular goiter, and I couldn't find a single study showing a correlation between stress and multinodular goiter.

IGF-1 and other thyroid stimulating factors. Numerous studies show that high amounts of insulin can result in an enlargement of various tissues and organs, including the thyroid gland. So high insulin levels can be a factor with both a goiter and thyroid nodules, and I mentioned this as a cause of thyroid nodules in Chapter 21. The insulin-like growth factor (IGF) system plays an important role in regulating normal development and growth of the thyroid and appears to be involved in thyroid cell hyperplasia.[270]

Estrogen dominance/problems with estrogen metabolism. I also mentioned this in Chapter 21 as a potential cause of thyroid nodules. It is well known that estrogen can promote the growth of certain types of cancer cells, but there is evidence that it can also be a potent growth factor for benign and malignant thyroid cells.[271, 272] While having high estrogen levels is an obvious sign of estrogen dominance, normal estrogen levels don't necessarily rule out estrogen dominance.

First of all, when evaluating blood work, I've seen a number of patients have normal, or even low estradiol/estrone levels, but high total estrogens. Second, if estrogen is normal but progesterone is low, then this is also considered to be a form of estrogen dominance. Finally, someone can have normal estrogen levels but an unequal distribution of the estrogen metabolites due to problems with phase 2 detoxification (specifically methylation, sulfation, and/or glutathione).

In other words, your body needs to detoxify estrogen, and if there is an impairment in one or more of the phase two detoxification pathways, then this can have a negative effect on estrogen metabolism. In Chapter 21 I also mentioned that there is a relationship between estrogen and the gut microbiome, and how having gut dysbiosis can cause problems with estrogen metabolism. And so improving the health of the gut microbiome can also play a role in having healthy estrogen metabolism.

So what happens is that as a result of one of the reasons I just mentioned, someone develops a multinodular goiter, which is initially non-toxic. But over a period of years there is a greater risk of the person with multinodular goiter developing hyperthyroidism. Toxic multinodular goiter can be associated with hyperfunctioning thyroid nodules (also known as toxic thyroid adenomas), which means that the nodules autonomously produces thyroid hormone. In fact, some sources consider ALL cases of toxic multinodular goiter to have nodules that produce thyroid hormone. Just in case this is confusing, there are a few different scenarios when someone has multinodular goiter in the presence of hyperthyroidism:

Scenario #1: Multinodular goiter with hyperthyroidism caused by nodules that produce thyroid hormone. Pretty much all sources consider this to be toxic multinodular goiter, while some label the other two scenarios I just mentioned as multinodular goiter in the presence of hyperthyroidism.

Scenario #2: Multinodular goiter with hyperthyroidism that isn't caused by nodules that produce thyroid hormone. Once again, some sources don't consider this to be toxic multinodular goiter, while other sources do.

Scenario #3: Multinodular goiter with hyperthyroidism caused by elevated thyroid stimulating immunoglobulins. This of course describes someone who has both multinodular goiter and Graves' disease.

Can an Iodine Deficiency Cause Toxic Multinodular Goiter?

There is evidence that in some cases an iodine deficiency relates to this condition, and one study I came across stated that the prevalence of nodular goiter is directly related to the degree of iodine deficiency.[273] The article goes on to state that "in iodine deficient areas such as some Italian regions, nodular goiter is present in 25-33% of the population, whereas in iodine sufficient areas the prevalence of nodular goiter is comprised between 0.4 and 7.2%, with the frequency increasing with age".

So does this mean that I recommend for everyone with a toxic multinodular goiter to take iodine? If you have read Chapter 13 you probably already know my response to this, as I do think iodine supplementation can be beneficial in some cases of multinodular goiter, but I would first focus on the other factors discussed, especially problems with estrogen metabolism and insulin resistance. And even if I were to recommend iodine supplementation I would first recommend a urinary iodine test to confirm that the person is deficient.

What Is The Conventional Treatment For a Toxic Multinodular Goiter?

Numerous studies show that a total thyroidectomy should be considered the procedure of choice for multinodular goiter.[274, 275] This is true even when someone has benign multinodular goiter.[276] Some medical doctors might not recommend surgery if someone has non-toxic multinodular goiter. However, a total thyroidectomy is used frequently for toxic multinodular goiter.[277]

One big concern with having a multinodular goiter is the risk of thyroid cancer. While the risk of thyroid cancer in people with this condition is relatively low, since it involves multiple thyroid nodules there might be an increased risk. One study looked to compare the thyroid cancer incidence in people with toxic and non-toxic multinodular goiter, and concluded that the incidence of malignancy in toxic multinodular goiter is not very low as thought earlier, and is nearly the same in non-toxic multinodular goiter.[278]

However, a more recent study looked at whether the prevalence of thyroid cancer is different in thyroid glands with a single nodule versus multinodular goiter.[279] It involved fourteen studies which included 23,565 patients with multinodular goiter, and 20,723 patients with a single nodule. The conclusion was that thyroid cancer might actually be less frequent in multinodular goiter, and this is especially true outside of the United States and possibly in iodine-deficient areas.

So does this mean that you shouldn't be concerned about thyroid cancer? There is always a concern, but just as is the case with everything else, one needs to look at both the risks and benefits. And while the risk of having thyroid cancer in people with a multinodular goiter is low, it still is possible.

However, there are risks with thyroid surgery itself, such as damage to the parathyroid glands and/or laryngeal nerve. And even if the surgery is successful, a total thyroidectomy will mean the person will need to take thyroid hormone replacement on a permanent basis. Once again, surgery is necessary for some people, but just as is the case with other hyperthyroid conditions, it usually should be a last resort, after more conservative treatments have been tried.

Address The Underlying Cause of Toxic Multinodular Goiter

It shouldn't be surprising that I recommend for people with toxic multinodular goiter to address the cause of their condition. While not everyone with this condition can be helped naturally, if someone has problems with estrogen metabolism, insulin resistance, or even an iodine deficiency, then it makes sense to address the cause of the problem before resorting to thyroid surgery. And even if natural treatment methods are unsuccessful, radiofrequency ablation might be an option to consider, which I discussed in Chapter 21.

In summary, most people who have a multinodular goiter can be helped naturally, although at times it can be a challenge. Sometimes it can be caused by an iodine deficiency, although problems with estrogen metabolism and insulin resistance are more likely causes, and should be looked into first. Either way, since conventional medical treatment usually involves a complete thyroidectomy, in many cases it is at least worth looking into a natural treatment approach.

Chapter Summary

- Multinodular goiter is characterized by a goiter, along with multiple thyroid nodules
- Toxic multinodular goiter involves an excess production of thyroid hormone, along with a goiter and multiple thyroid nodules
- Two common causes of a toxic multinodular goiter are 1) problems with estrogen metabolism and 2) insulin resistance
- There is evidence that in some cases an iodine deficiency can cause a multinodular goiter
- The conventional medical treatment for a multinodular goiter is a thyroidectomy
- If addressing the cause of the problem doesn't restore the health of someone with toxic multinodular goiter, before getting surgery you might want to consider radiofrequency ablation

For access to the book references and resources, visit
savemythyroid.com/hyperbooknotes

CHAPTER 26

5 Reasons Why You Shouldn't Self-Treat Your Hyperthyroid Condition

AFTER GOING THROUGH a couple of consultations and receiving my recommendations, Keesha figured that she could correct her hyperthyroid condition on her own. She went ahead and changed her diet, purchased some supplements and herbs, and put together her own natural treatment protocol. At first she began feeling better, as the bugleweed and motherwort she was taking helped to improve her symptoms. But when she received her follow-up blood tests two months later the lab values had worsened. She decided to continue self-treating her condition, and after a couple of months passed by the lab values improved. She was ecstatic, and since she was feeling much better she decided to wean herself off of the antithyroid medication she was taking.

She had completely weaned herself off the medication, but a few months later she began experiencing some palpitations again, and when she had more follow-up blood tests they had worsened again. At this point Keesha wasn't sure what she should do. Should she take the antithyroid medication again? Or should she try taking different supplements and herbs?

She finally decided to stop self-treating her condition, as our office received an email from her stating that she was ready to follow my recommendations. She did have to take the antithyroid medication again temporarily, but a few months after following my recommendations she eventually weaned herself off the medication (her own decision of course), while still taking the bugleweed and motherwort, and she continuously got better, and eventually her symptoms resolved and blood tests normalized.

Many people with hyperthyroidism don't want to manage their symptoms by taking antithyroid medication, and most people want to avoid receiving radioactive iodine treatment if at all possible. This is great, as these people realize there is an underlying cause behind their problem, and they want to attempt treating their condition naturally. Chances are this is why you are reading this book.

Of course some people do need to take antithyroid medication, and some people do need to get thyroid surgery. But as I've mentioned already throughout this book, many people with hyperthyroidism can restore their health, and many of these people attempt to do so on their own. As a result, they gather as much information as they can through reading books and surfing the internet, and then attempt to find and remove their triggers and underlying imbalances without the help of a natural healthcare practitioner.

Sometimes people will see positive changes in their symptoms when self-treating their hyperthyroid condition. But most people who attempt to self-treat their condition aren't able to fully restore their health. So I decided to dedicate this chapter to those people who are looking to take a natural approach, but are thinking about self-treating their condition.

What I'm going to do next is list five reasons why you shouldn't self-treat your condition. This is true whether you have Graves' disease or a non-autoimmune hyperthyroid condition.

Reason #1: There are risks when self-treating your condition. Even when using natural supplements and herbs, there are always risks involved. Most people don't have a strong knowledge of these supplements and herbs, and many assume that because they are natural there is no risk involved. While the risk might be minimal, it still exists. Plus, just abruptly stopping any antithyroid medication you may be taking and replacing these prescription drugs with nutritional supplements and herbs makes it even more risky.

This doesn't mean that you can't get some improvements with diet and lifestyle. And some people will experience dramatic changes by improving their diet, improving their stress handling skills, etc. But while I encourage you to do things to improve your diet and lifestyle, usually you will need to go beyond diet and lifestyle in order to restore your health.

Reason #2: You can't trust everything you read and listen to. Once again, many people try to restore their health based on what they read in a book, or have viewed on the internet. Heck, some people try to piece the information I provide on my website or podcast to find and remove their triggers, correct other underlying imbalances, etc. Of course different people will need to take different supplements and herbs, and will also require different dosages. As a result, it's extremely difficult to come up with a treatment plan which will work based on the information you read on my website, my podcast, this book, or anywhere else.

And a lot of the information on "natural cures" put out there is by people who don't have much experience with this. Many aren't even healthcare professionals. This doesn't mean there aren't people who are very knowledgeable about natural treatments. You just need to be extremely careful about any information you read on the internet, videos you watch on YouTube, etc.

Reason #3: The body is extremely complex. Although it would be great if one could restore their health simply by eating well and taking some supplements and herbs, in most cases it isn't this easy. Obviously eating well and taking supplements and/or herbs is very important to restore one's health. But doing this alone usually won't restore your health, even though it might allow you to feel better initially. But if you're looking to completely regain your health, just remember that the body is very complex, and because of this it is highly unlikely you will receive optimal results by self-treating your condition.

Reason #4: It probably will cost you more money in the long run. Many people choose to self-treat their condition because they figure they will save money by taking this approach. After all, they won't need to pay a natural healthcare practitioner for an initial consultation or any follow-up visits. And I completely understand, as it's expensive to work with an experienced natural healthcare practitioner, especially since it takes time to restore one's health.

And obviously I'm biased because I'm a natural healthcare practitioner. Once again, if you want to see how much your health will improve by changing your diet and lifestyle that's fine, but you want to make sure you safely manage your hyperthyroid symptoms while doing this. And if your health doesn't improve I would urge you to work with an expert, as while you might save money initially when self-treating your condition, in the end it almost always will cost you more money.

Reason #5: You most likely won't receive optimal results. This obviously relates to the previous four reasons I just spoke about, as for all of the reasons I have mentioned, it is unlikely you will receive optimal results by self-treating your condition naturally. Once again, this doesn't mean that you can't experience some positive changes by improving your diet and lifestyle. In fact, since writing the first edition of this book in 2011 I've gotten emails from people who have felt a lot better by following the advice given in this book. On the other hand, many people won't receive optimal results when self-treating their condition, which of course is the purpose behind this chapter.

In summary, while it might seem easy enough to self-treat your condition, the truth is that for the reasons I've mentioned in this chapter, most people don't receive optimal results when taking this approach. This is why I dedicate a chapter in this book on consulting with a natural healthcare professional who focuses on thyroid and autoimmune thyroid conditions, as anyone who is serious about restoring their health should speak with an expert. While there still isn't any guarantee by taking this approach, you stand a much better chance of restoring your health than if you were to attempt this on your own.

Chapter Summary

- Sometimes people will see positive changes in their symptoms when self-treating their hyperthyroid condition. But most people who attempt to self-treat their condition aren't able to successfully restore their health.
- Most people don't have a strong knowledge of these supplements and herbs, and many assume that because they are natural there is no risk involved. While the risk might be minimal, it still exists.
- Different people will need to take different supplements and herbs, and will also require different dosages. As a result, it's extremely difficult to come up with a treatment plan which will work based on the information you read on my website, this book, or anywhere else.
- While you might save money initially by self-treating your condition, in the end it almost always will cost you more money when taking this approach.

For access to the book references and resources, visit
savemythyroid.com/hyperbooknotes

CHAPTER 27

Natural Treatment Methods Don't Cure Anything

EVEN THOUGH I HAVE mentioned the word "cure" a few times in this book, the truth is that natural treatment methods really don't cure anything, as it's the person's body which needs to take all of the credit. I'll explain more about this shortly, but before I do this I want to remind you that in Chapter 6, where I discussed the difference between a cure and a remission I admitted that I honestly don't know whether anybody with hyperthyroidism who takes a natural treatment approach can be permanently cured. And as I also discussed, I think that most people would be fine knowing that their condition can't be completely cured, as long as they were able to maintain a good state of health and avoid taking antithyroid drugs or receive radioactive iodine treatment.

After all, the overall goal is to get you to the point where you are able to visit an endocrinologist, or any medical doctor for that matter, and test completely negative for a hyperthyroid condition. In other words, after taking a natural treatment approach, the goal is that if you were to visit an endocrinologist and if you got tested for hyperthyroidism, ideally EVERY test you received would be negative. So in addition to having a normal TSH and thyroid hormone levels, someone with Graves' disease should also test negative for thyroid antibodies.

In addition, other tests should eventually normalize as well. For example, I commonly recommend adrenal testing to my patients, and of course want to eventually see normal results on this test. If someone has positive findings on a comprehensive stool panel then these should also greatly improve. And the same is true for any other tests I might recommend. Of course one can't rely on tests alone, which is why it's extremely difficult to tell whether someone is ever truly cured or not. This is why I usually use the words "restoring one's health", rather than "curing your condition".

What The Real Goal Of A Natural Treatment Approach Is

In any case, when I recommend a natural treatment approach to a patient, I am telling them to do things which will assist their body in the healing process. Many other healthcare practitioners take the same approach. For example, I have a chiropractic degree, and when I had my chiropractic practice and saw people with neck pain, back pain, and other similar conditions, the goal wasn't necessarily to "cure" the back pain condition. In fact, in chiropractic college chiropractors aren't trained to cure anything, as they are taught to deal with spinal subluxations, which are misalignments in the spine which cause nerve interference. This in turn can lead to conditions such as neck pain, back pain, but it can also lead to other health issues as well.

So when someone who is experiencing back pain visits a chiropractor, obviously the chiropractor will want to try relieving the person's pain. But although this is the main reason the person decided to schedule an appointment in the first place, the chiropractor's primary goal isn't to provide pain relief, but is to determine whether there is a spinal subluxation which is causing or contributing to the person's pain, and then correct this spinal subluxation. While correcting the subluxation will frequently eliminate the person's back pain, one needs to also remember that the nerves of the spine supply every organ and tissue in the body.

As a result, it's possible that this nerve interference can not only cause back pain, but can lead to other health issues. For example, if the nerve that is being affected is supplying the kidney, then this in turn can cause kidney problems. If there is a spinal subluxation which is affecting the nerve supplying the thyroid gland, then this can cause or contribute to a thyroid condition as well.

How Does This Relate To Taking A Natural Treatment Approach To Hyperthyroidism?

My point here is not to convince you to see a chiropractor, but instead is to reveal to you how most natural healthcare practitioners are interested in helping the individual achieve optimal health by giving the body what it needs to self-heal. So when someone goes to a chiropractor with neck or back pain, a good chiropractor will focus on the patient's desires, which is to get relief from their pain. But they will also try to help them achieve optimal spinal health. Similarly, when someone who has hyperthyroidism consults with me, or any other thyroid condition, my goal is not to treat and cure the condition, but is to give the person what they need to help their body achieve optimal health.

So when I tell someone to eat well, get sufficient sleep, do a better job of managing their stress, and to take certain nutritional supplements and/ or herbs, I don't do this in order to "cure" their condition. I do this in order to help them regain their health. Some people think the nutritional supplements and/or herbs they take are used to cure their condition, but these supplements and/or herbs are recommended to assist the compromised body.

For example, someone who has severe adrenal imbalances might be able to restore their health by modifying certain lifestyle factors. However, certain supplements and herbs can usually help to assist in the recovery process. Similarly, if someone has a disrupted gut microbiota then they might need to take supplements and herbs to help rebalance the intestinal flora and repair the gut. The same concept applies with addressing the compromised immune system, as I frequently recommend certain supplements and herbs to help with this.

But as I've mentioned before, if someone is successful in restoring their health but then begins eating junk food frequently, neglects their sleep, and gets stressed out all of the time, there is an excellent chance that over time they will suffer a relapse. Or perhaps they won't develop hyperthyroidism again, but instead will develop a different condition. Either way, any good natural healthcare practitioner won't only try to help a person achieve optimal health, but will also give the person the information and guidance they need to maintain their health.

The Dentistry Model Provides A Good Example Of Preventative Maintenance

If you want to look at a good model of preventative maintenance, then look no further than your local dentist. Most dentists will not only fill cavities, extract teeth, and perform other dental procedures, but they will also teach the patient how they can maintain healthy teeth. This of course involves brushing one's teeth two or three times each day, flossing daily, and visiting your dentist twice each year for regular checkups and cleanings.

However, if someone restores their oral health, but stops brushing their teeth, or perhaps only brushes their teeth every now and then, doesn't floss, and doesn't go to the dentist regularly, then there is a good chance that over time they will develop dental problems.

As difficult as it is to take a natural treatment approach and restore one's health, it's also challenging to maintain one's health. But as I frequently tell people, after you have restored your health it's not necessary to live a perfect lifestyle in order to maintain your health. If you eat some junk food every now and then, get stressed out once in awhile, and get only five or six hours of quality sleep once or twice each month, then this most likely won't cause a relapse to occur. If your body is healthy and strong, then it will do a great job of adapting to "acute" stress situations. It's the chronic stress, or frequent bad habits your body can't deal with.

In summary, the goal of this book, as well as my website and podcast, isn't to provide you with information to help cure your hyperthyroidism. And when someone chooses me as their healthcare provider and I consult with them, I'm also not trying to cure anything. I'm just giving them the information and tools necessary for them to achieve optimal health. So for those people who get their health restored back to normal due to my advice, don't thank me, but instead thank your wonderful self-healing body.

Chapter Summary

- Even though I do mention the word "cure" at times in this book, the truth is that natural treatment methods really don't cure anything, as it's the person's body which needs to take all of the credit.
- When I recommend a natural treatment approach to a patient, I am telling them to do things which will assist their body in the healing process.
- Some people think the nutritional supplements and herbs they take are used to cure their condition, but they are recommended to assist in the healing process.
- As difficult as it is to take a natural treatment approach and restore one's health, it's also challenging to maintain a state of wellness.

For access to the book references and resources, visit
savemythyroid.com/hyperbooknotes

CHAPTER 28

What Can You Do If Natural Treatment Methods Aren't Effective?

ALTHOUGH I WISH I CAN say that everyone with a hyperthyroid condition who takes a natural treatment approach will receive great results, the truth is that some people don't respond as expected. Most of the time this is due to the person not completely following my recommendations. But sometimes the person will follow the recommendations and still not receive optimal results. When this is the case then you need to consider the following options:

1. **Make sure you're following the recommendations.** If you're not responding as expected, then you want to make sure you're following the complete recommendations. For example, if you are told to eat mostly whole foods, and avoid common allergens such as gluten, dairy, and corn, then you need to ask yourself if you are following these recommendations. Sometimes a person will think they are following the recommendations, but aren't aware that they are inadvertently cheating.

For example, many people are sensitive to corn. But most people aren't aware that ascorbic acid, which is sold in most health food stores as Vitamin C, is derived from corn. As a result, a person may think they're avoiding corn because they're not eating any foods which contain corn, but they might not be aware that some of their supplements include corn, even if this isn't mentioned on the label. Or if they go out to eat there very well might be cross contamination, and as a result they might get exposed to gluten.

Another example relates with managing your stress levels. I've had patients who did a wonderful job of eating well and avoiding common allergens, and also took all of the nutritional supplements I recommended, but didn't do a good job of managing their stress. Remember that the adrenals respond to stress by secreting cortisol, and if cortisol is constantly being secreted then this is going to lead to all sorts of problems. And so besides eating well and taking nutritional supplements you need to manage your stress levels. Similarly, you also need to make sure you get sufficient sleep each night.

2. **Look at the adrenals, gut, and toxic burden.** As you know by now, there are many different factors which can lead to the development of hyperthyroidism. But I have found that three of the most important factors to look at are 1) the health of your adrenals, 2) the health of your gut, and 3) your toxic burden. With the adrenals, hopefully you understand the importance of testing through the saliva or dried urine. The reason for this is because you want to look at the cortisol levels throughout the day.

Some people assume that their adrenals are fine because they don't feel fatigued and/or don't have problems with sleep. While many people with adrenal problems experience fatigue and/or sleeping difficulties, keep in mind that when I was diagnosed with Graves' disease I felt fine from an energy standpoint and also had no problem falling or staying asleep. However, my cortisol levels and DHEA were extremely depressed. So you can't go by symptoms alone when evaluating the health of your adrenals.

The same concept applies with the gut, as while many people with gut problems experience symptoms such as bloating, gas, and/or bowel irregularities (i.e. constipation or diarrhea), some people with gut problems don't have any digestive symptoms. In fact, I've had many people have positive findings on a comprehensive stool panel, even though they felt fine from a symptomatic standpoint. And when they do things to improve the health of their gut microbiome, in most cases their health improves dramatically. There's a reason why most natural healthcare professionals focus a great deal on the health of the gut, and the reason is because if someone has an unhealthy gut, then it is not possible to achieve optimal health.

As for environmental toxins, since dealing with Graves' disease I've always been an advocate of doing things to reduce one's toxic load by minimizing one's exposure to environmental toxins and doing things to support the elimination of them from your body. Obviously nothing is going to completely eliminate the toxins from one's body. However, in addition to eating well and taking certain detoxification supplements, some people need to utilize other procedures such as colon hydrotherapy and colonic irrigation, as well as infrared sauna. So if you're not responding to a natural treatment approach, environmental toxins could very well be the reason, as sometimes just eating well and taking nutritional supplements isn't sufficient.

3. **Consult with a different natural healthcare practitioner.** If you have taken a natural treatment approach and haven't received good results, consider seeing a different natural healthcare professional. If the person you

worked with isn't someone who focuses on thyroid and autoimmune thyroid conditions, then you might want to consider consulting with someone who focuses on these problems. It doesn't matter which type of natural healthcare practitioner you see, as long as they have experience dealing with hyperthyroidism.

This might mean driving a few hours to see the person, or speaking with someone remotely over the phone or through Zoom. While some people are fortunate to have a practitioner in their town who has experience helping people with hyperthyroid conditions, some people aren't as lucky. Either way, if you've seen a single natural healthcare practitioner and didn't receive ideal results, consider getting a second, and perhaps even third opinion before resorting to RAI or thyroid surgery.

4. **Consider low dose naltrexone (LDN).** Naltrexone is a prescription medication, and it was originally approved by the FDA as a treatment for heroin and opium addicts, as it blocks the effects of these drugs. 50mg was the typical dosage used for this, but in 1985, Dr. Bernard Bihari discovered that lower dosages of naltrexone helped to enhance the person's immune system.

Fast forward to today, and LDN is used to help people with different types of conditions in order to modulate the immune system. This includes HIV, cancer, Parkinson's disease, and autoimmune conditions, including Graves' disease and Hashimoto's thyroiditis. I've had patients with Graves' disease and Hashimoto's who received great results when taking LDN. On the other hand, I've also had patients take it and not see any positive changes in their symptoms or blood tests.

With regards to research studies, there are some studies which demonstrate the benefits of LDN.[280, 281] Although there aren't any specific studies I know of which show whether LDN can help people with Graves' disease, there are a few studies which have shown the benefits of LDN and multiple sclerosis,[282, 283] which is a different type of autoimmune condition. I also came across some research which showed that LDN reduces the need for medication used in the treatment of rheumatoid and seropositive arthritis.[284]

How Can Low Dose Naltrexone Help?

This drug blocks the opiate receptors, which increases the levels of endorphins, and this in turn will modulate the immune system. This can sometimes result in a reduction of thyroid antibodies. So the goal is to restore the body's levels of endorphins, which is commonly depleted in people with autoimmune thyroid conditions, and doing this will essentially help to suppress the autoimmune response in people with Graves' disease and Hashimoto's.

What Are The Pros and Cons of LDN?

The benefits of taking LDN are that it potentially can suppress the auto-immune response, thus lowering the thyroid antibodies, and eliminate the person's symptoms. It also is relatively inexpensive. Since the dosage is very small (usually around 1 to 5 mg) side effects are rare. These are three good reasons to consider giving this treatment a try.

However, there are some disadvantages to this treatment. One disadvantage is that that not everyone who takes LDN will respond. Another downside is that the person will need to take this medication for the rest of their life if they don't do anything to address the underlying cause. Of course if it doesn't cause any long term side effects then this might not be a problem. And while it doesn't seem to have immediate side effects, the long term effects are still unknown.

The biggest problem with relying on LDN alone is that it still doesn't address the underlying cause of the condition. Yes, it may help to control the autoimmune response in those with Graves' disease, which is causing the thyroid gland to secrete an excessive amount of thyroid hormone. But it won't do anything for the cause of the autoimmune condition.

In other words, taking LDN won't address the factor or factors which triggered the autoimmune response in the first place, which is why you will need to take it on a permanent basis if you relied on it alone. So it will do absolutely nothing for compromised adrenal glands, vitamin and mineral deficiencies, a leaky gut, toxic metals, imbalances of the sex hormones, etc. While it might be a better option than receiving radioactive iodine treatment or getting your thyroid gland surgically removed, LDN is not a cure for Graves' disease, or any other autoimmune condition.

Combining LDN With A Natural Treatment Approach

I'm not opposed to people with Graves' disease taking LDN. However, for those people who choose LDN I recommend combining it with a natural treatment approach. Even though LDN doesn't seem to have any serious side effects, I'm still not thrilled about people taking any type of medication on a long term basis, and so I would of course prefer for someone to take a natural treatment approach alone at first, and then perhaps incorporate LDN later on if the person isn't responding as expected.

5. **Consider long-term treatment with methimazole or bugleweed.** In countries outside of the United States, many endocrinologists will do everything they can to help their patients avoid RAI and thyroid surgery. It's not uncommon for them to recommend long-term treatment with low doses of antithyroid medication, such as methimazole. In fact, there have been a couple of studies which compared long-term continuous use of methimazole with RAI.

One study that was conducted concluded that long-term continuous treatment of hyperthyroidism with methimazole is safe. It also concluded that the complications and the expense of giving methimazole long-term do not exceed those of radioactive iodine therapy.[285] A second study came to the conclusion that long-term methimazole treatment was superior to RAI therapy in patients when mood, cognition, cardiac function and occurrence of thyroid dysfunction were compared.[286]

Although I'm not thrilled about people taking any prescription drug on a long term basis, remember that we're comparing risks vs. benefits. Plus, most people who receive RAI or thyroid surgery will be taking thyroid hormone for the rest of their life. It's almost a "no win" situation, but in my opinion everything should be done to preserve the health of the thyroid gland. And while some people will be sensitive to even low doses of methimazole, for most people it won't be a problem taking a low dose (i.e. 5 mg/day).

What should you do if you bring this up to your endocrinologist and he or she isn't supportive of long-term treatment with methimazole? Well, this is where you need to take a stand. And so I would be firm, but at the same time polite, and if you're unable to talk your endocrinologist into letting you take low doses of methimazole on a long term basis, then I would speak with a different endocrinologist. And don't be afraid to show them the research which demonstrates the safety of long-term treatment with methimazole, which you can check out by visiting savemythyroid.com/hyperbooknotes.

Another option is to take low doses of bugleweed on a long-term basis to manage your symptoms. Once again, this isn't the ideal situation, as I was able to wean off of bugleweed for good, and most of my patients who are on bugleweed are also eventually able to stop taking this herb. Of course I would recommend for people to consult with a natural healthcare professional if they're considering taking bugleweed for a prolonged period of time.

For some people, taking low doses of methimazole or bugleweed won't be sufficient to manage the symptoms. When this is the case LDN should be considered, although another option is cholestyramine, which I'll discuss next.

6. **Consider cholestyramine.** Cholestyramine is a bile acid sequestrant. It binds to certain components of bile, which in turn disrupts the entero-hepatic circulation of bile acids. Bile acid sequestrants are commonly used for lowering cholesterol or for the treatment of chronic diarrhea (when the cause is due to bile acid malabsorption). Cholestyramine can also bind to mycotoxins, and thus can be used as a treatment for toxic mold, although it of course is also important to remove the source of the mold.

Cholestyramine has been shown to interfere with the enterohepatic circulation of endogenous thyroid hormones, which is increased in hyperthyroidism.[287] Simply put, it binds to thyroid hormones and then the hormones are excreted by the body.

What Does The Research Show?

One study evaluated the efficacy and safety of high-dose cholestyramine added to antithyroid medication in order to control hyperthyroidism.[288] This was a small study, involving only five patients, all who took at least 30 mg of methimazole. They were put on 4 grams of cholestyramine three times a day for four weeks. When compared to a control group consisting of patients who only took methimazole, the group who took both the methimazole and cholestyramine showed a more rapid reduction of the T3 and T4 levels in nearly all subjects.

In another study, this one a randomized, double-blind, placebo-controlled trial involving 45 patients newly diagnosed with Graves' disease, the patients were randomly assigned into three treatment protocols.[289] Group one took 2 grams of cholestyramine twice per day, group two took one gram of cholestyramine twice per day, and group three took a placebo powder. All three groups took 30 mg of methimazole and 40 mg of propranolol each day. The length of the study was 4 weeks, and the thyroid hormone levels decreased more rapidly and to a greater extent in the cholestyramine-treated groups. In addition, all of the patients in group one had normal thyroid hormone levels at the end of the study.

These studies, along with a few case reports,[290, 291] showed that cholestyramine can decrease thyroid hormone levels more rapidly when combined with methimazole. But how about if cholestyramine is taken without any antithyroid medication? I was able to find a case report involving a 36-year old woman who was diagnosed with Graves' disease, and was unable to take antithyroid medication due to side effects.[292] Four grams of cholestyramine was given every six hours, and while unfortunately the woman ended up receiving radioactive iodine, prior to receiving this treatment her free T4 levels improved significantly within five days. Although this is only a single case study, it did provide some evidence that cholestyramine might be an effective monotherapy for those with hyperthyroidism who are unable to take antithyroid medication.

I can't say that I've had a lot of patients with hyperthyroidism take cholestyramine, but it has been effective when it has been taken. And all of the cases I've seen involved people taking cholestyramine without antithyroid medication. The main downside is that it comes in a powder form and doesn't taste good, plus it needs to be taken away from food and supplements. But if someone is unable to take antithyroid medication and the natural agents don't work, then it's something to consider. If you do ask your endocrinologist about this I would make sure to show him or her the research studies, which will be included in the references at savemythyroid. com/hyperbooknotes

Choosing Between Radioactive Iodine Treatment And Thyroid Surgery

When I consult with a patient, I will do everything I can to prevent them from receiving RAI or a thyroidectomy. However, I don't have a 100% success rate and so every now and then someone will need to choose between these two treatment methods. So what I'd like to do is discuss the benefits and risks of RAI and thyroid surgery.

Benefits of Radioactive Iodine Treatment: One of the main reasons I wrote this book is because I'm not a big fan of radioactive iodine, and so it admittedly will be difficult to prevent my biases from getting in the way here. But as much as I don't like radioactive iodine, it can help to eliminate the hyperthyroid symptoms in many people. Plus when all goes well, the hypothyroid symptoms that are likely to develop can usually be managed by taking thyroid hormone. And RAI isn't as invasive as surgery, as RAI can be taken orally. So the treatment procedure itself is painless, and you aren't subjected to the risks of surgery, which I'll describe shortly.

Risks of Radioactive Iodine Treatment. Where should I start? How about the fact that you are putting something into your body that has radiation? You may not think this is too big of a deal, as we're all exposed to small amounts of radiation throughout our lives. An example involves getting x-rays.

However, when you get one or more x-rays you aren't given special instructions which involve flushing the toilet multiple times after going to the bathroom, not being intimate with your spouse, and in some countries they still quarantine people for a few days who receive RAI. So while I'm not suggesting that receiving radioactive iodine treatment will lead to the health issues I described in Chapter 18, one still can't dismiss the potential effects this treatment will have on your body.

In addition to the radiation exposure, the goal of radioactive iodine treatment is to make you hypothyroid. And while many people just take thyroid hormone replacement and live happily ever after, for some people it isn't this simple. Some people don't do well on either synthetic or natural thyroid hormone, even after the dose has been adjusted multiple times.

In addition, I have received emails from some people who received RAI who experienced other symptoms that aren't typical of hypothyroidism. Whether these symptoms were the result of the radiation I honestly don't know, but it's rare that I get the same complaint from someone who has received a thyroidectomy. So another downside is that the person might feel worse after getting RAI, and most endocrinologists don't know what to do when this happens, other than trying to change the dosage of thyroid hormone, or just telling the person to live with the symptoms.

Finally, radioactive iodine treatment does nothing for the actual cause of the condition. So for example, Graves' disease is an autoimmune condition in which thyroid stimulating immunoglobulins attack the TSH receptors and cause excess secretion of thyroid hormone. Something is triggering the autoimmune response, as it could be a certain food, chronic stress, an infection or environmental toxin, etc.

Either way, receiving RAI will obliterate the thyroid gland, thus helping with the excessive secretion of thyroid hormone. But it won't do anything to stop the autoimmune response, won't correct compromised adrenal glands, dysbiosis of the gut, address nutrient deficiencies, etc. Perhaps this is one of the reasons why many people who receive RAI don't do well, even when taking thyroid hormone. In these cases the thyroid hormone they're taking might be helping, but perhaps these other compromised areas are causing or contributing to their symptoms.

Benefits of Receiving a Thyroidectomy. The main "benefit" of receiving a thyroidectomy in someone with a hyperthyroid condition is that you no longer have to worry about the thyroid gland secreting an excessive amount of thyroid hormone. And unlike RAI, thyroid surgery doesn't involve any radiation, and a second thyroid surgery is usually not required for those who receive a complete thyroidectomy. I mention this because some people will need multiple treatments with RAI, whereas when someone receives a complete thyroidectomy there is just about no doubt that it will eliminate the hyperthyroid symptoms, since there is no thyroid gland to produce any thyroid hormone. While no surgery is completely safe, most people who receive thyroid surgery do fine, and this is especially true if they choose a surgeon with a good amount of experience, which I discussed in Chapter 21.

While most surgeons will recommend a complete thyroidectomy, sometimes a partial thyroidectomy is an option. Although some people who have their thyroid gland partially removed will still need to take thyroid hormone daily for the rest of their life, some people won't need to take thyroid hormone. So this is an option to consider, especially if someone has a single toxic nodule, although radiofrequency ablation is another option to consider, which I discussed in Chapter 21.

Risks of Receiving a Thyroidectomy. As is the case with any surgery, there are risks associated with surgery of the thyroid gland. There is the risk of damage to some of the surrounding structures, such as the laryngeal nerve, and the parathyroid glands. Of course a definite consequence of a complete thyroidectomy is that the person will need to take either synthetic or natural thyroid hormone for the rest of their life.

And as I mentioned earlier, there are some people who just don't seem to do well when taking thyroid hormone. At least with radioactive iodine there's a very small chance that it will result in the person becoming euthyroid, where they no longer experience hyperthyroid symptoms, but also don't experience hypothyroidism.

Just as is the case with RAI, a big disadvantage of a thyroidectomy is that it does absolutely nothing for the underlying cause of the condition. Once again, it is rare for the thyroid gland to be the actual cause of the condition. And when this is the case, removing the thyroid gland won't do anything to correct other compromised areas of the body.

Which Treatment Option Should You Choose?

So now that you know both the benefits and risks of RAI and a thyroidectomy, if you happen to be faced with choosing one of these two treatment options, then which one should you choose? I obviously can't make this decision for you. Although I hope my Graves' disease condition will continue to stay in remission for the rest of my days, if I absolutely had to choose between these two treatment options, I'm pretty sure I would choose thyroid surgery. Of course I realize it's easy for me to say this when I'm not in this situation, and perhaps I would choose RAI, although I don't think I would.

That being said, if I did choose a thyroidectomy I would make sure to find an experienced surgeon, even if it meant driving to another city or state. But I understand that this isn't an easy decision to make, and so when someone sends me an email, or posts a comment in one of my Facebook groups telling me that they have received radioactive iodine treatment, I never criticize them for this decision. After all, while some people regret their decision to receive RAI, others feel it was one of the best decisions they ever made.

In summary, while my goal is to try to restore people's health naturally so they don't need to receive RAI or thyroid surgery, there of course are times when these conventional medical treatment methods are necessary. And I hope those people who need to choose between radioactive iodine and thyroid surgery will find this information to be helpful in making their decision. But before resorting to these treatment methods, please consider the other suggestions given in this chapter.

Chapter Summary

- If someone follows the recommended natural treatment protocol and don't receive optimal results then they need to consider the following options: 1) make sure you're following the recommended protocol, 2) look at the gut, adrenals, and toxins, 3) consult with a different natural healthcare professional, 4) consider low dose naltrexone (LDN), 5) consider cholestyramine, 6) consider long-term treatment with methimazole or bugleweed
- Although LDN can potentially suppress the autoimmune response, not everyone who takes it will respond. In addition, it doesn't address the cause of the condition, which means that if it does work the person will most likely need to take it for the rest of their life.
- If someone needs to choose between radioactive iodine treatment and thyroid surgery, they need to carefully look at the benefits and risks of each procedure before making a decision.

For access to the book references and resources, visit
savemythyroid.com/hyperbooknotes

CHAPTER 29

The Keys To Maintaining Your Health

MANDY WAS DOING GREAT following my recommendations for her Graves' disease condition, as her hyperthyroid symptoms subsided after only a few months, and eventually her test results normalized. Things were going great, and I went ahead and began weaning her off most of the supplements and herbs, and recommended a wellness protocol. It consisted of a few basic nutritional supplements, and of course I encouraged her to continue eating well, manage her stress, etc.

However, Mandy's grandmother became very ill, and being that she was close to her grandmother this was very stressful. She tried her best to manage the stress, but had a difficult time doing so. And due to everything that was going on she also began eating poorly. Eventually the hyperthyroid symptoms returned, and unfortunately the blood tests revealed that her Graves' disease had returned.

For those people who have restored their health by taking a natural treatment approach, the obvious goal is to maintain their health. While maintaining a state of wellness is usually easier than restoring one's health, it still can be a challenge for people to maintain their health, and thus prevent a relapse from occurring. I was hesitant to include a negative story at the beginning of this chapter, as I don't want people to think that relapses are common whenever a stressful situation comes along, or that eating some junk food every now and then after restoring your health will cause a relapse to occur. As of writing the third edition of this book I have maintained a state of wellness since 2009, even though I've had plenty of stressful events and don't live a perfect lifestyle. And the same can be said for many of my patients who have taken a natural treatment approach.

As you know, in order to restore your health from a hyperthyroid condition, it is necessary to eat well, get sufficient sleep, manage your stress, minimize your exposure to environmental toxins, take certain nutritional supplements and/or herbs, etc. Although one usually doesn't need to take such extreme measures when maintaining a state of wellness, it's still important to take responsibility for your health.

The Two Most Difficult Lifestyle Factors To Manage

After restoring one's health, I find that for most people, the two most challenging lifestyle factors to keep up with are eating well and doing a good job of managing stress. With regards to eating well, it's important to understand that you don't need to healthy 100% of the time in order to maintain a state of wellness. So it's a different story than when trying to restore your health, as you know that while healing you should eat only whole healthy foods, while avoiding the refined foods and sugars, along with avoiding common allergens such as gluten and dairy.

After one has restored their health, it's still important to eat mostly whole foods and minimize the amount of refined foods and sugars. But this doesn't mean that someone can't indulge in some "bad" foods every now and then. I admit that I indulge every now and then. While I eat well most of the time, every now and then I will eat foods that are considered to be unhealthy.

For example, there are times when my family and I will go out for pizza at a local pizza place, or we'll get some dessert (chocolate chip cookies, ice cream, etc.). Of course this isn't what I do on a regular basis, as once again, I do eat healthy most of the time. I should add that I still try to eat gluten free when I indulge, and so if I have pizza it's usually with a cauliflower crust, and if I have dessert I also usually stick with gluten free options.

Of course when I initially took a natural treatment approach I didn't eat any of these "bad" foods, and it wasn't easy to avoid pizza, cookies, etc. But back to my current situation, I'd be lying if I told you that I didn't go out occasionally and eat foods that aren't considered to be healthy. For most people who have already restored their health, indulging every now and then isn't too big of a deal.

Of course there are exceptions to this. I've mentioned earlier in this book that someone who has Celiac disease shouldn't eat gluten-based foods every now and then. On the other hand, some natural healthcare professionals tell all of their patients with autoimmune conditions such as Graves' disease that they need to permanently avoid gluten-based foods. While I can't say that I've been 100% gluten free since 2009, I mentioned before how I usually try to avoid gluten, although I eat dairy a little more frequently. For example, if I were to eat out and order a cauliflower crust pizza, even if they have dairy-free cheeses available I always opt for mozzarella cheese!

Try Not To Get Stressed Out

In addition to maintaining a healthy diet, it's also important to continue doing a good job of managing your stress. Just as is the case with eating healthy, if you get stressed out every now and then it probably won't lead to a relapse. On the other hand, if you let stress get the best of you frequently then there is a good chance you will become symptomatic again.

As I mentioned in Chapter 8, I would block out at least five minutes per day for stress management, and once you're in the routine continue doing at least five minutes per day, but perhaps a few days per week you can do 10 to 15 minutes per day. The stress management technique you choose to do isn't as important, and as I also briefly mentioned in Chapter 8, I use a type of biofeedback device called the Inner Balance, which is from the company HeartMath.

The Inner Balance measures heart rate variability (HRV), which is the variation in time interval between heartbeats, and is a measurement of autonomic nervous system function. A healthy heart is supposed to have a greater amount of variability in between the heart beats. Heart rate is regulated by the sympathetic and parasympathetic nervous systems, which are part of the autonomic nervous system. Having higher HRV is a sign of good adaptation and characterizes a person with efficient autonomic mechanisms, while having a lower HRV is usually an indicator of abnormal and insufficient adaptation of the autonomic nervous system.[293]

I probably should add that most of my patients don't use HeartMath as their form of stress management. Incorporating other mind body medicine techniques such as yoga and meditation is fine. I'm just mentioning HeartMath here because I know that some people will be interested in the methods I use for stress management.

Which Nutritional Supplements Should You Take To Maintain Your Health?

After someone restores their health they won't need to take as many supplements as they were taking while addressing their triggers and underlying imbalances. In most cases they will just need to take some basic supplements to maintain their health. Here are some of the supplements I currently take on a regular basis for wellness purposes:

1. **Probiotic supplement.** I've been taking a probiotic supplement for many years, and I recommend for my patients to do the same after they have restored their health. If you eat fermented foods on a daily basis then perhaps you don't need to take a daily probiotic supplement, although you need to keep in mind that you will get different strains in a probiotic than you would in fermented foods, and the more variety of strains you're exposed to the better. I'll add that I don't take the same probiotic supplement every day, as I rotate my probiotic supplements.

2. **Prebiotics.** These are a more recent addition, as I add a prebiotic powder to my daily smoothie. I specifically add prebiotic inulin and acacia fiber. Since I add this to my smoothie I honestly don't look at this as a typical supplement, and the prebiotics I currently use are very cost effective. To check out the prebiotics I currently take, along with other supplements, visit savemythyroid.com/ hyperbooknotes.

3. **Omega-3 Fatty Acids.** Most people can also benefit from taking omega 3 fatty acids daily, along with a good source of GLA (i.e. Black Currant seed oil, Borage oil, etc.). With regards to omega 3 fatty acids I take a fish oil supplement, and you can check the quality of the supplement by cutting one of the softgels open to make sure they don't have a fishy smell, which means that it's rancid. How about flax seeds? Although I grind a tablespoon of whole flaxseeds and add it to my smoothie,

I also take fish oils, and the reason is because Alpha-linolenic acid (ALA), which is the parent fatty acid found in flaxseed oil, needs to be converted to EPA and DHA. And studies have shown that many people have problems with this conversion. [294] On the other hand, fish oils already have EPA and DHA, and so you don't have to worry about the conversion process.

4. **Multivitamin.** This is another recent edition, as over the years I've gone back and forth when it comes to taking a daily multivitamin. And when taking it I don't always take the full dosage, as I might take half the recommended dosage.

5. **Vitamin D3.** One of the things I'm guilty of is not getting enough sun, although I am doing a better job now than I was when I wrote the first and second editions of this book. That being said, I still take 5,000 IU/day of vitamin D3 (with vitamin K2) to maintain levels above 50 ng/ml.

6. **Magnesium.** I've been taking a magnesium supplement for many years, as this mineral has many important functions in the body. Of course I also try to get magnesium from the food I eat.

7. **Methylation supplement.** I don't recommend for everyone to take a methylation supplement, but in Chapter 12 I mentioned that in the past I had an elevated homocysteine marker, and then I did genetic testing, which showed I had a homozygous MTHFR C677T genetic polymorphism. Although I don't recommend genetic testing to everyone with hyperthyroidism, if this is something you're interested in you can visit savemythyroid.com/ hyperbooknotes to see what companies I recommend.

8. **Digestive enzymes.** Years ago I took digestive enzymes on a daily basis, but these days I just take them on an as-needed basis. For example, if

I eat a larger meal that is very high in protein I might take a digestive enzyme, but I can't say I take them routinely with each meal.

9. **Electrolytes.** Since doing sauna therapy I have been taking electrolytes, which I mix in a glass of purified water, but more recently I started taking electrolytes on a daily basis. If you want to see which electrolytes I use you can visit savemythyroid.com/hyperbooknotes.

Another Key Lifestyle Factor: Getting Sufficient Sleep

I've already discussed the importance of getting proper sleep in this book, but since it's so important for optimal health I'll bring it up again here. Not only is getting sufficient sleep essential when it comes to restoring one's health, but it also is important for maintaining a state of wellness. So while eating well and stress management are essential, so is getting quality sleep each night.

I've been pretty good about getting a good night's sleep for most of my life, as while I can't say that I never stay up late, it's rare that I stay up past 10:30 these days. And more recently I've been going to bed between 9:30 and 10pm. I'm sure some people reading this think there is no way they can go to bed this early, while others might go to bed even earlier than I do. If you're in the latter category then I'd like to commend you for going to bed super early, and if you're a night owl I want to let you know that you can change your habits, but it probably will take some time before you are routinely going to bed earlier.

Continue To Reduce Your Toxic Burden

In Chapter 14 I discussed the impact of environmental toxins, and so I'm not going to get into great detail here. But I do think that continuously working on reducing my toxic load has also played a big role in maintaining a state of wellness. Of course you want to do as much as you can through food, especially by eating plenty of vegetables.

In addition to having smoothies on most days, a few times per year I do a prolonged detoxification program involving supplements that support the liver, bile, kidneys, etc. In addition, I do infrared sauna two to three times per week. As I mentioned in Chapter 14, I would be cautious about doing sauna if you have unmanaged hyperthyroidism, but in this chapter I'm focusing on what you can do to maintain a state of wellness. One more thing I should add is that I didn't start doing sauna therapy until approximately five years after being in remission from Graves' disease, and so please don't think that you need to do sauna in order to maintain a state of wellness.

In summary, while restoring your health can be challenging, it also isn't easy to maintain one's health. However, this doesn't mean that people who have restored their health need to live a perfect lifestyle and eat a perfect diet. While some people have food allergies and sensitivities which prohibit them from eating certain foods, most people who restore their health can indulge every now and then. Also remember that you want to work on stress management on a daily basis, try to get sufficient sleep each night, etc.

Chapter Summary

- For those people who have restored their health back to normal naturally, maintaining a state of wellness can be a challenge.
- After restoring one's health, for most people the two most difficult lifestyle factors to keep up with are eating well and doing a good job of managing stress.
- Upon restoring one's health, one doesn't need to eat a perfect diet, but they should still eat mostly whole foods and minimize the refined foods and sugars.
- While maintaining a state of wellness you shouldn't have to take a lot of supplements.

For access to the book references and resources, visit
savemythyroid.com/hyperbooknotes

CHAPTER 30

Consult With A Natural
Healthcare Practitioner

WHEN APRIL WAS INITIALLY diagnosed with Graves' disease, she wanted to get to the underlying cause of the problem. So she called a local functional medicine doctor and scheduled an appointment for a consultation. April wasn't sure if the doctor had much experience with Graves' disease, but there weren't too many other options, as she preferred to speak with someone face-to-face, and so she figured she would have nothing to lose by giving this doctor a try. The functional medicine doctor put her on a specific diet and advised her to take certain supplements and herbs. April followed the recommendations for two months, but she didn't notice much of an improvement with her symptoms.

April viewed one of my free webinars, and she then scheduled an appointment to speak with me. I told her that I would welcome the opportunity to help her, but at the same time I suggested for her to give the other functional medicine doctor a fair chance to help her. After all, while many of my patients experience positive changes quickly, this isn't the case with everyone. And even though the functional medicine doctor she was working with didn't focus on thyroid conditions, I told her she probably should give his recommendations a little more time.

April followed this doctor's recommendations for two additional months, still didn't see much of an improvement in her symptoms, or any significant changes with her follow-up blood tests. At that point I agreed to work with her, she did some additional testing, and about five weeks after she began following my recommendations she began noticing a reduction in her symptoms, positive changes in her thyroid blood tests after two months, and eventually her symptoms were completely gone and her thyroid blood tests normalized.

If you have hyperthyroidism and want to address the underlying cause of your condition, then you will most likely want to consult with a natural healthcare practitioner who focuses on thyroid and autoimmune thyroid conditions such as hyperthyroidism and Graves' disease. However, finding such a person can be a challenge. You of course can choose to speak with a "general" functional medicine practitioner, and sometimes you can receive good results if you choose your practitioner wisely.

However, being someone who personally dealt with Graves' disease and successfully used a natural treatment approach to restore my health, for optimal results I strongly recommend speaking with a natural healthcare practitioner who focuses on thyroid health. There are numerous medical doctors, naturopaths, and chiropractors who focus on thyroid and autoimmune thyroid conditions.

But how do you find a competent natural healthcare practitioner who focuses on thyroid and autoimmune thyroid conditions? Well, one way is through a referral, as if you know someone who happened to be treated by a such a practitioner and received great results, then this is definitely someone who you will want to contact. Of course many people don't have such a connection, and so they resort to searching for a natural healthcare practitioner on their own. This definitely can be a challenge.

What's even more challenging is that many natural healthcare practitioners don't want anything to do with hyperthyroidism. While many healthcare professionals have a lot of experience with patients who have hypothyroidism and Hashimoto's thyroiditis, since the symptoms of hyperthyroidism can be scary, and even life threatening at times, many don't want to take the risk of treating hyperthyroidism naturally. And many healthcare professionals who are willing to help people with hyperthyroidism will insist for them to take antithyroid drugs to manage the symptoms. As you know, there is a time and place for antithyroid medication, but there are some people who prefer to manage their symptoms naturally like I did when I dealt with Graves' disease.

How To Find A Local Practitioner Who Focuses On Thyroid Health

If you can't get referred to such a practitioner by a friend or family member who has seen one, then there are a few options you have. You of course can perform an online search for a natural healthcare practitioner, followed by the state and city you live in. This will give you an opportunity to visit their website to see if they really focus on thyroid and autoimmune thyroid conditions.

If you can't find anyone by conducting an online search, then another option is to put together a list of all of the natural healthcare practitioners within a 50 mile radius of where you live. This should include naturopathic doctors, chiropractors, and medical doctors who practice functional medicine. If you're not willing to drive this far then make it a 25 mile radius, or if you're willing to drive further then perhaps you'll want to make it a 100 mile radius. In any case, begin calling these offices. Chances are you'll get the front desk receptionist, and when you do, make sure you ask the following question:

"What are the top three conditions the doctor commonly sees?"

If one of the top three conditions isn't thyroid and/or autoimmune thyroid conditions, then it's time to move onto the next office. If they give a response such as "the doctor sees people with all types of conditions", then once again you should move onto the next office. I'm not suggesting that a general practitioner can't help restore the health of someone with hyperthyroidism, but it is best to consult with someone who has a good deal of experience dealing with these conditions.

Better yet, before you begin calling these offices, you might want to visit the websites of these natural healthcare practitioners. And then whenever you come across a website that focuses on thyroid conditions go ahead and jot this down. Keep in mind that some offices have multiple websites for different conditions, and so even if you find a website that claims the doctor specializes in thyroid or autoimmune thyroid conditions, it still is a good idea to call them and ask the question regarding the top three conditions the doctor deals with.

Working With a Natural Healthcare Practitioner Remotely

While it would be great if you can find a thyroid expert who practices close to where you live or work so that you can see them in person, the good news is that you usually don't need to speak with a natural healthcare practitioner face-to-face in order to receive great results. Assuming you have already been diagnosed with hyperthyroidism by an endocrinologist or general medical practitioner, and received a physical examination, then in most cases it's perfectly fine to consult with a doctor remotely over the phone or through Zoom.

In fact, phone and Zoom consultations are a routine part of my practice, and this was even the case before the pandemic. Since there aren't a lot of natural healthcare professionals who focus on hyperthyroidism, most of the people I consult with live in different states, and I also speak with people internationally as well. In some cases people were able to visit a local natural healthcare professional, but they preferred to speak with someone who has a lot of experience with hyperthyroidism.

Plus, I'm sure it also helps that I personally dealt with my own Graves' disease condition and have been in remission since 2009 after taking a natural treatment approach. Because of this, people with this condition know I could relate with them. But there are many other natural healthcare practitioners who conduct phone and Zoom consultations, especially since the pandemic in 2020.

There are some nice benefits of working with a practitioner remotely. One big advantage is not having to wait in a doctor's office way past your appointment time. Plus, it's nice to speak from the comfort of your own home, or even at work during your lunch break without having to take time off. Plus, you don't have to drive to an office, pay extra money for fuel, deal with rush hour traffic, etc. So convenience is definitely one of the benefits of speaking with a natural healthcare professional remotely.

Using The Internet To Find A Natural Healthcare Practitioner

As I mentioned before, you of course can also use the internet to search for a natural healthcare professional that focuses on helping those with thyroid and autoimmune thyroid conditions. You do need to be careful, as there are some practitioners who might claim they specialize in thyroid health, when the truth is that they accept many other types of cases, and as a result only deal with a handful of hyperthyroid patients on a monthly, or even an annual basis. This doesn't mean you need to consult with a practitioner who has seen hundreds or thousands of people with hyperthyroidism, but it is a good idea to see someone who has seen a fair share of people with these conditions.

Getting back to searching on the web, you of course can visit your favorite search engine and type in the words "Natural Endocrine Doctor" or "Natural Thyroid Specialist", followed by the name of the city you live in, and then call some of the doctors listed as I mentioned before to determine which one might be a good fit for you. I do give a few resources in my free guide entitled "The 6 Steps On How To Treat Graves' disease & Hashimoto's thyroiditis Through Natural Methods". If you haven't received your free copy you can get it simply by visiting my website at naturalendocrinesolutions.com and then just enter your name and email address.

Speaking With Someone Who Doesn't Focus On Thyroid Health

Can you receive good results from a natural healthcare practitioner who doesn't focus their practice on thyroid health? For example, if there is a local naturopathic physician, chiropractor, or medical doctor who practices functional medicine in your area, is it possible to receive great results under the care of such a doctor, even if they don't have much experience dealing with thyroid and autoimmune thyroid conditions? Of course it is possible, as there are healthcare professionals who don't focus on thyroid health, yet still have some experience helping people with hyperthyroidism. The problem is that you don't know who these people are, as it's easy for anyone to tell you they have experience, but it's difficult to know if they are telling the truth.

For example, while numerous chiropractors like myself focus on thyroid health, most chiropractors don't focus on such conditions. So if you were to randomly call some of the local chiropractors in your area, there is a good chance that none of them will have much experience helping people with hyperthyroidism. There is a better chance that a local naturopathic physician will have had some experience seeing some hyperthyroid patients, but then again, there is also the chance they might not have a lot of experience seeing people with hyperthyroidism. In fact, with some natural healthcare practitioners you would be their very first person presenting with hyperthyroidism.

As I've already mentioned, a good way of finding out whether a natural healthcare practitioner focuses on thyroid health is to visit their website. If you visit their website and they have many different health conditions listed, then you know that they don't focus on thyroid and autoimmune thyroid conditions. Once again, this doesn't mean they don't have experience dealing with hyperthyroidism.

On the other hand, if their website only focuses on thyroid and autoimmune thyroid conditions, AND if they have been in practice for awhile, then you can be confident that they have a good deal of experience seeing people with conditions similar to yours. Then again, there are some doctors who have a "niche" website for different conditions to make it look like they specialize in certain areas. In other words, they might have a separate website for thyroid conditions, another one for digestive disorders, etc.

I'm not going to advise you not to see a "general" natural healthcare practitioner, as in most cases this obviously is a better option than receiving radioactive iodine or thyroid surgery. But if you have a choice between seeing a general natural healthcare professional and one who focuses on thyroid health, then it's obviously better to see someone who has dealt with a lot of people with hyperthyroidism. On the other hand, just because someone focuses on thyroid health doesn't mean they have dealt with a large number of people with these conditions, as perhaps they mainly have dealt with hypothyroid conditions, and maybe even focus their practice on other conditions such as diabetes, women fertility issues, etc.

I Repeat, Self-Treating Your Condition Can Be Risky

One of the reasons why some people with hyperthyroidism choose to self-treat their condition is due to the challenge of finding a competent natural healthcare practitioner. As I've already discussed in a previous chapter, I'm not a fan of self-treating any thyroid or autoimmune thyroid condition naturally, but it's especially unwise to treat hyperthyroidism on your own. So once again, please don't self-treat your condition, as in most cases these conditions are too complex to successfully self-treat on your own.

In summary, finding a competent natural healthcare practitioner who focuses on thyroid health can be a challenge, but if you want to receive optimal results then you should consider speaking with someone who focuses their practice on thyroid and autoimmune thyroid conditions. While it may be tempting to self-treat your condition, for optimal results it's wise to consult with an expert.

Chapter Summary

- If you have hyperthyroidism and want to use natural treatment methods to restore your health back to normal, then you will most likely want to consult with a natural healthcare practitioner who focuses on thyroid and autoimmune thyroid conditions.
- Some natural healthcare practitioners don't want anything to do with hyperthyroidism, which can make it challenging to find someone to help treat your condition naturally.
- Assuming you've already been diagnosed with hyperthyroidism by an endocrinologist or general medical practitioner, and have received a physical examination, then in most cases it's perfectly fine to consult with a doctor remotely over the phone or through Zoom or Skype.
- You do need to be careful, as there are some doctors who might claim they specialize in thyroid health but who only deal with a handful of hyperthyroid patients on a monthly or annual basis.

For access to the book references and resources, visit
savemythyroid.com/hyperbooknotes

CHAPTER 31

Formulate An Action Plan
To Restore Your Health

Now that you're just about done reading this book, I hope you are convinced that you should at least consider taking a natural treatment approach. Just about everyone with hyperthyroidism are told by their endocrinologist that there is no choice but to take antithyroid drugs for a prolonged period of time, or to receive radioactive iodine treatment or thyroid surgery. But you now have the information required to potentially restore your health, and to help you achieve optimal health in all other areas of your life as well.

What I'd like to do is help you to design an action plan to restore your health. While restoring your health isn't an easy process, if you're willing to take responsibility for your health then not only can you restore your health, but you probably will feel much better than you have in years. Much of this chapter will be a summary of what you have read in this book, and in order to help keep you motivated I recommend reviewing this chapter on a weekly basis until you have gone through these steps.

Here are four action steps you can take:

Action Step #1: Have A Natural Mindset. Chances are you already have a natural mindset if you're reading this book, but even if you're not fully convinced that natural treatment methods can restore your health, this doesn't mean you still can't have a natural mindset. Obviously you know that your hyperthyroid condition didn't develop due to a deficiency of antithyroid drugs or radioactive iodine. Something caused this condition to develop, and therefore for most people the goal should be to find the cause of the condition, rather than just manage the symptoms.

Action Step #2: Modify Certain Diet and Lifestyle Factors. Hopefully you've already made some diet and lifestyle changes, but if not I would start doing so immediately, as this is a key factor in restoring your health. For example, if you're currently eating a lot of refined foods and sugars, then make it a goal to incorporate more whole foods into your diet. In fact, you can take it to a different level and completely eliminate any processed foods or sugars for at least 30 days, drink half your weight in ounces of purified water daily (or spring water out of a glass bottle), and then see how you feel. Just keep in mind that even if you don't notice an improvement in your symptoms, this doesn't mean that improving your diet and lifestyle isn't benefiting your health. It just means that there are other factors that need to be addressed.

A good next step would be to try to eliminate common food allergens such as gluten, dairy, and corn. Try to eat as many organic foods as possible, and try to avoid genetically modified foods, which includes most corn and soy. Eventually work to get your daily carbohydrate intake below 200 grams per day, which shouldn't be too difficult if you are focusing on eating healthier carbohydrates. Make sure you also eat a sufficient amount of protein each day, which I discussed in Chapter 11.

In addition to eating well, try to get at least seven to eight hours of sleep each night, and some people need more than this while healing. Also, don't forget the importance of stress management, as I would block out at least five minutes per day to get into the routine of blocking out time for stress management. Refer to Chapter 8 for more information on this. Even if you eat well and get sufficient sleep, if you remain stressed out and do a poor job of handling the stress then you will never achieve optimal health. Modifying these lifestyle factors really can do wonders for your health.

With regards to supplements, ideally you should consult with a natural healthcare practitioner before taking herbs such as bugleweed and motherwort, along with some of the other supplements and herbs I discussed in Chapter 12. But you probably can take some basic supplements on your own, such as a good quality probiotic that has well-researched strains, along with an omega-3 fatty acid supplement. I usually just start my patients with a few basic supplements, and then recommend some testing to see what else they need to take to support their adrenals, correct nutrient deficiencies, etc.

Action Step #3: Do Everything You Can To Avoid RAI and Thyroid Surgery. By reading this book you are obviously motivated to avoid radioactive iodine and thyroid surgery. But reading this book alone won't be sufficient, as you need to take action, which is the purpose of this chapter!

Some endocrinologists will tell their patients with hyperthyroidism that radioactive iodine is the only option. Others will tell you that it is the best option. Most of the time RAI should be the last resort. I can't tell you not to receive radioactive iodine, as this is ultimately a decision you will need to make on your own. But I will encourage you to avoid it if at all possible.

RAI is never the "only option", as one can always choose to receive a thyroidectomy, which in some cases might be a better option. But obviously the goal of this book is to not only prevent you from receiving radioactive iodine, but also to prevent you from having your thyroid gland surgically removed.

Before you receive radioactive iodine or thyroid surgery, just remember that neither of these treatment methods will do anything for the underlying cause of the condition. Approximately 90% of hyperthyroid conditions are autoimmune, and so receiving RAI or thyroid surgery won't do anything to help restore the health of the immune system, and of course won't do anything to remove the triggers which are responsible for the autoimmune response.

And of course conventional medical treatment won't address other compromised areas of the body, such as the adrenals, digestive system, and the sex hormones. For those who don't have Graves' disease, RAI and thyroid surgery also won't do anything for the cause of their condition. Once again, this doesn't mean these conventional treatment methods are never required, and hopefully the information in this book will help you to weight the benefits and risks so you can make an informed decision.

Action Step #4: Find Your Triggers and Underlying Imbalances. Chances are you chose to read this book because you wanted to try to avoid conventional medical treatment, especially radioactive iodine and thyroid surgery. If you're like most people reading this book, then you're interested in restoring your health, but before reading this book you were probably skeptical about both the safety and effectiveness of natural treatment methods. At this point you still might be skeptical, but hopefully reading this book has at least convinced you to give natural treatment methods a try.

For those people who choose to receive radioactive iodine treatment or thyroid surgery, I at least want them to be 100% comfortable with their decision. While some people go through these procedures and do fine, each week I receive numerous emails from people who received these treatment methods and regretted their decision. Many at least wish they had given natural treatment methods a try before receiving radioactive iodine treatment or thyroid surgery. So whatever treatment option you choose, I don't want you to have any regrets.

As you know, if you choose to take a natural treatment approach then I would advise you to consult with a natural healthcare professional who focuses on thyroid and autoimmune thyroid conditions. Some people feel I say this in order to promote my services. The truth is that I don't care whether someone consults with me or another healthcare professional. After all, I'm not the only healthcare professional who focuses on thyroid and autoimmune thyroid conditions, and if you're persistent you probably will find one who practices close to where you live or work.

But the reason why you want to work with someone is because it can be challenging to detect and remove the trigger or triggers which caused your hyperthyroid condition to develop, and it is also a challenge to restore the health of other compromised areas of the body. Because of this, you definitely don't want to self-treat your condition, and working with an expert will greatly improve your chances of receiving optimal results.

So these are four action steps you can take to help restore your health. While it is without question a challenge for anyone with hyperthyroidism to restore their health, most people willing to make such a commitment will find it well worth it to take a natural treatment approach. The problem is that most people aren't willing to take responsibility for their health, and as a result they will choose to live with their condition, or eventually receive radioactive iodine or thyroid surgery and take thyroid hormone on a permanent basis.

That being said, I'd like to thank you for reading this book. I hope you found the information to be valuable, and if so, I do hope that you will take action. In the next chapter I will discuss some additional resources you can check out to learn more about natural thyroid health.

Chapter Summary

- Even if you're not fully convinced that natural treatment methods can restore your health back to normal, this doesn't mean you still can't have a natural mindset.
- Chances are you can make some lifestyle changes which can cause a significant improvement in your condition.
- I can't tell anyone not to receive radioactive iodine, as this is ultimately a decision each individual with hyperthyroidism will need to make on their own. But in most cases it should be the last resort.
- As mentioned in the previous chapter, while you can see a "general" holistic doctor, in my opinion it makes sense to consult with someone who has a great deal of experience dealing with thyroid and autoimmune thyroid conditions.

For access to the book references and resources, visit
savemythyroid.com/hyperbooknotes

CHAPTER 32

Additional Natural Thyroid Health Resources

IF YOU ENJOYED READING this book, I highly recommend checking out some of the resources listed in this chapter, most of which are free.

Resources related to this book. As I've mentioned after each of the chapter summaries, you can access all of the book references and resources by visiting savemythyroid.com/hyperbooknotes.

Save My Thyroid Podcast. This podcast has been out since the summer of 2021, and while many of the episodes can benefit those with both hyperthyroidism and Hashimoto's thyroiditis, if you skim through the episodes you'll notice that there definitely is an emphasis on hyperthyroidism. You can check out the Save My Thyroid podcast by visiting your favorite podcast platform, or you can listen by visiting savemythyroid.com/podcast and you can also access the show notes to each episode on this website.

Thyroid/Immune Health Restoration Checklist. This is a comprehensive checklist that includes 12 action points you can take to find and remove your autoimmune thyroid triggers. You can access this free checklist by visiting savemythyroidchecklist.com.

Natural Endocrine Solutions website. I created this website in 2010, and there are hundreds of articles and blog posts, many of which focus on hyperthyroidism. You'll notice that more recently that most of the blog posts are transcripts of the podcast episodes, although there are also many articles and blog posts that are unique, which you can easily find by using the search bar. For example, if you wanted to see what blog posts I've written on bugleweed you can enter the keyword "bugleweed" and it will pull up any related articles.

When you visit www.naturalendocrinesolutions.com you can also check out my free guide, which is entitled "The 6 Steps On How To Treat Hyperthyroidism and Graves' disease Through Natural Methods". Just to let you know, in order to obtain the free guide I do require people to submit their name and email address, which not only gives you access to this free guide, but will also give you email updates whenever I release a new blog post or podcast episode. There are no catches to obtaining this free guide, and of course you are always welcome to cancel your email subscription at any time.

Free Recorded Webinar on Hyperthyroidism. This recorded webinar is entitled "5 Steps To Reverse Hyperthyroidism and Avoid Radioactive Iodine and Thyroid Surgery". The first 35 minutes consists of pure content, and then I discuss my program for those with hyperthyroidism. In fact, before anyone works with me I require them to watch this so that they can know what to expect. You can check this recorded webinar by visiting savemythyroid. com/hyperwebinar.

Hyperthyroid Healing Community: I also have a couple of thyroid-related communities you might want to join, but one specific to hyperthyroidism is called "Graves Disease & Hyperthyroidism: Natural Treatment Solutions", and you can join this by visiting savemythyroid.com/community. As of writing this third edition of the book there are over 10,000 members, and it's a great place to connect with others who are also dealing with hyperthyroidism.

YouTube Channel. The name of my YouTube channel is Natural Thyroid Doctor, and most of the recent videos are actually interviews I did on my podcast, and repurposed into YouTube videos. But there are some other videos that don't involve any interviews.

Save My Thyroid Quiz. Find out what you need to do to save your thyroid by taking the "Thyroid Saving Score" quiz. Once you complete the quiz you will receive a free report explaining your results. You can take the quiz by visiting savemythyroidquiz.com.

Foundations of Overcoming Hyperthyroidism Online Course. This free online course will discuss the basics you need to overcome your hyperthyroid condition. To learn more about this visit savemythyroid.com/foundations.

Hyperthyroid Healing Diet book. Of course this isn't a free resource, but it is a very low cost one. I'm writing this third edition in 2023, and the plan is for my next book to be released in the first quarter of 2024. If I hadn't already started on the book this would probably be wishful thinking, but I actually have a lot of the book already written, and so it's not unrealistic for it to be released within the first quarter of 2024.

Interested in working with me? If you want to do everything to save your thyroid and are interested in working with my team and I, visit workwithdreric.com.

CHAPTER 33

Twenty Three Questions You May Have

Question #1: Should Gluten Be Completely Avoided In People With Hyperthyroidism & Graves' Disease?

There is a lot of controversy involving gluten consumption in people with autoimmune conditions such as Graves' disease. Although I do eat gluten free most of the time, I can't say that I've been 100% gluten free since being in remission in 2009. I don't feel bad when I eat gluten, but I still know that it's inflammatory and can have a negative effect on the permeability of the gut.

Currently I recommend for my patients to avoid gluten while trying to restore their health, regardless of whether or not they experience symptoms when consuming gluten. Testing for a gluten sensitivity is an option, although the problem is that testing for a gluten sensitivity problem isn't completely accurate. And keep in mind that if you obtained a Celiac panel and it came out negative this doesn't confirm that you're not sensitive to gluten.

Question #2: Can a Goiter Be Decreased In People With Hyperthyroidism & Graves' Disease?

Goiter is a condition that is characterized by an enlargement of the thyroid gland. In people with hyperthyroidism it is usually caused by the overproduction of thyroid hormone, although it can also be caused by a malignancy, problems with estrogen metabolism, insulin resistance, or an iodine deficiency. The typical goiter treatment consists of treating the hyperthyroidism through antithyroid drugs, radioactive iodine, or thyroid surgery. The latter is usually indicated if the person has an obstruction that is causing difficulty in swallowing and/or breathing.

When a goiter is caused by an excess production of thyroid hormone, problems with estrogen metabolism, insulin resistance, or an iodine deficiency, then many times it's possible to correct this problem through a natural treatment approach. When I was initially diagnosed with Graves' disease I had a small goiter, and at times it caused difficulty swallowing. This resolved after I took a natural treatment approach. Sometimes a larger goiter won't respond as well to natural treatment methods. Other times the goiter will decrease, but won't completely resolve. This is especially true for very large goiters.

Question #3: What's The Difference Between Radioactive Iodine and Radiofrequency Ablation?

Radioactive iodine is a treatment method that obliterates the cells of the thyroid gland. So radioactive iodine essentially damages the thyroid gland, and most people who receive this treatment will need to take thyroid hormone replacement. On the other hand, as I discussed in Chapter 21, the goal of radiofrequency ablation is to preserve the thyroid gland by removing thyroid nodules. So if someone has one or more thyroid nodules and radioactive iodine is recommended, they might want to first consider radiofrequency ablation.

Question #4: I Took Bugleweed For My Hyperthyroid Symptoms And It Didn't Help. Can You Explain Why?

Although bugleweed will help many people with hyperthyroidism, there are some people who take it and don't notice much of a change in their symptoms or thyroid hormone levels. First of all, remember that it can take a few weeks before beginning to experience a decrease in the hyperthyroid symptoms after taking bugleweed. In some people it can take up to four weeks before noticing a difference, although most people should notice a decrease in their symptoms sooner than this. Also, keep in mind that someone who has severe hyperthyroid symptoms might not be able to have their symptoms managed by taking bugleweed alone. Sometimes taking larger doses of L-carnitine tartrate (i.e. 2,000 mg to 4,000 mg/day) can help, but some people will need to take antithyroid medication to manage the symptoms.

Question #5: What Should I Do If I Can't Tolerate Antithyroid Medication and Natural Agents Aren't Effective?

Over the years I've had a good number of patients who were sensitive to antithyroid medication, and therefore were told by their endocrinologist that they will need to receive radioactive iodine or thyroid surgery. First of all, just because someone is sensitive to methimazole doesn't mean they will also have a negative reaction to PTU. So if someone is sensitive to methimazole, for example, then they might be able to take PTU, and vice versa. Keep in mind while the main dangers are with the cardiac symptoms, such as the high pulse rate, elevated thyroid hormones can also have a negative effect on bone density. If someone is unable to tolerate both methimazole and PTU, and if natural agents such as bugleweed and L-carnitine aren't effective, then one option is to take a beta blocker such as propanolol. This not only will help with the cardiac symptoms, but can also inhibit the conversion of T4 to T3. Two other options are to take low dose naltrexone (LDN) or cholestyramine, which I discussed in Chapter 28. It ultimately is up to the patient as to what they decide to do, as my goal is not to talk someone out of receiving radioactive iodine or thyroid surgery, but is once again to present them with the different options they have so they can make an informed decision, and not feel as if they're being pressured by their endocrinologist to receive radioactive iodine or thyroid surgery.

Question #6: Can Natural Treatment Methods Help People With Subclinical Hyperthyroidism?

Just as is the case with overt hyperthyroidism, many people with subclinical hyperthyroidism can be helped naturally. That being said, sometimes it can be more challenging to help these people, mainly because the TSH is the only lab value which is usually out of range, and they are experiencing minimal symptoms when first consulting with them. As a result, it could be difficult to tell whether someone is responding to a natural treatment approach from a symptomatic standpoint. Obviously one shouldn't rely on symptoms alone, but symptoms are still important in monitoring a person's response to a natural treatment approach. In people with subclinical hyperthyroidism it is even more important to look at other tests such as an adrenal saliva test or comprehensive stool panel, so they can clearly see that they have other positive findings, and not just a depressed TSH.

Question #7: Can People With Hyperthyroidism Exercise Regularly?

I'm all for regular exercise and keeping fit, but people with hyperthyroid conditions do need to be cautious when exercising. This is especially true if someone has a high pulse rate. This doesn't mean that people with hyperthyroidism can't exercise, as I do think it's important to be active. I typically limit my patients with hyperthyroid conditions to walking while taking a natural treatment approach, and I think some resistance exercise can also be beneficial to help increase muscle mass and bone density, both of which are usually affected in hyperthyroidism. I know it can be difficult to refrain from vigorous exercise, but you don't want to overexert yourself, as this can exacerbate your condition.

Question #8: Can Iodine Cause The Development Of An Autoimmune Thyroid Condition?

There is some evidence that taking iodine can trigger an autoimmune response, thus leading to a condition such as Graves' disease. Once again, iodine is a controversial topic, and just as a reminder, when I wrote the first two editions of this book I was frequently recommending iodine testing and supplements to my patients with hyperthyroidism, and I personally had a good experience with iodine supplementation. That being said, iodine can also trigger or exacerbate thyroid autoimmunity in some people, which is why I've been more cautious with iodine recently. But as I discussed in this book, I don't recommend to completely avoid foods that have iodine, and if I recommend a multivitamin I think that in most cases it's fine to take one that has iodine. But I usually advise against taking separate iodine supplements, and I'm also cautious when it comes to eating foods that are extremely high in iodine, such as sea vegetables.

Question #9: Do You Have Any Advice For Picky Eaters When It Comes To Taking A Natural Treatment Approach?

Even though I eat pretty healthy now, I have always considered myself to be a picky eater. I grew up eating cold cereal for breakfast, hamburgers, spaghetti, plenty of canned foods, cookies and cakes, soda and punch, etc. I rarely ate vegetables growing up, and as a result I've never been a vegetable lover, which is why I rely a lot on smoothies. I never ate organic food growing up, never went to a health food store until I went to chiropractic college, and I was always hesitant to try new foods. Even to this day I can't say I eat a wide variety of foods.

However, I am a lot better than I was in the past, and the best advice I can give to picky eaters is to slowly start changing your eating habits. If you're living off of fast food and hate eating vegetables, I don't expect you to immediately begin eating five servings of vegetables each day. If this is the case I would begin with one serving of vegetables per day, and then try to add one additional serving each week. You also might want to look into different types of seasonings to help make the taste of vegetables more appealing, or do what I do and make a daily smoothie. I should add that while I do have smoothies on a daily basis, I also eat some vegetables other than the ones I add to my smoothie.

Question #10: Can Someone Have Both Graves' Disease and Hashimoto's Thyroiditis At The Same Time?

It is possible to have the antibodies for both Graves' disease and Hashimoto's thyroiditis at the same time. As a result, a person can fluctuate back and forth between hyperthyroidism and hypothyroidism, although this isn't too common. What more commonly happens is that the person will start out with hyperthyroidism, but if nothing is done to address the autoimmune component then they eventually might become hypothyroid. That being said, I've also worked with people who were once hypothyroid but then eventually became hyperthyroid. Either way the goal is to find and remove triggers and correct underlying imbalances, although the symptom management aspect will of course differ if someone has hyperthyroidism vs. hypothyroidism.

Question #11: What Effect Does Alcohol Have On Thyroid Health?

Although some sources claim that drinking a lot of alcoholic beverages can depress the activity of the thyroid gland, thus resulting in a hypothyroid condition, the main effects of excess alcohol consumption is on the liver, gut, and adrenal glands. Just remember that alcohol is a carbohydrate and will affect the blood sugar levels, and thus consuming a lot of alcohol over a period of months and years can compromise the adrenals. In addition, alcohol can increase the permeability of the gut. Does this mean that someone who takes a natural treatment approach and drinks an alcoholic beverage on a frequent basis won't receive optimal results? Once again, it depends on the person, as if someone already has compromised adrenals, a leaky gut, or a liver that isn't detoxifying properly, then having one or two alcoholic beverages per week might be too much, let alone one or two per day. But to play it safe I usually advise people to avoid alcohol while taking a natural treatment approach.

Question #12: Can A Vegetarian Receive Good Results When Taking A Natural Treatment Approach?

One of the main challenges of being a vegetarian or vegan is consuming enough protein. If you happen to be a pescatarian then this won't be as challenging, but if you're a strict vegetarian or vegan then you will need to rely on other sources. Following an AIP diet can be very challenging for a strict vegan or vegetarian. If you're a vegetarian then you can always follow a standard Paleo diet and get some of your protein from eggs. On the other hand, if you're a vegan then you may have no choice but to eat some properly prepared legumes. Speaking of which, many vegetarians will get a lot of their protein from soy, and while I do think there are some good health benefits of organic, fermented soy, since soy is a common allergen I usually recommend for people to avoid it while restoring their health.

Question #13: I Thought Most People With Hyperthyroidism Lose Weight. Why Am I Gaining Weight?

Although most people with hyperthyroidism do in fact lose weight, some people with hyperthyroidism gain weight. This frequently occurs when taking the antithyroid medication, which of course decreases thyroid hormone production, and can potentially lead to weight gain. However, some people with hyperthyroidism will gain wait, even if they aren't taking antithyroid medication. There can be a few different reasons for this, including high cortisol, insulin resistance, estrogen dominance, an increased toxic load, and even widespread inflammation can make it very difficult to lose weight.

Question #14: Can Hyperthyroidism Affect The Sex Hormones?

It is common for hyperthyroidism to cause imbalances of the sex hormones. For a woman in premenopause, this might cause her to stop cycling, although sometimes it will result in shorter cycles. It's also important to mention that healthy adrenals are important for healthy sex hormones, and many people with hyperthyroidism have compromised adrenals. And so while there is a time and place for bioidentical hormones, I think it's important to first optimize the health of the thyroid and adrenals.

If the sex hormones are still low after balancing the thyroid hormones and optimizing the health of your adrenals then perhaps you should consider taking bioidentical hormones. So while I do think there is a time and place for bioidentical hormones, this doesn't mean that everyone who has low sex hormones should take them.

Question #15: Will I Increase My Risk Of Developing Atrial Fibrillation By Taking A Natural Treatment Approach?

Atrial fibrillation is the most common cardiac arrhythmia other than sinus tachycardia encountered in hyperthyroidism, and it occurs in 10-15% of patients with hyperthyroidism.[178] This definitely is a concern, but the key is to effectively manage the hyperthyroid symptoms, which I have discussed in this book. This can be accomplished through the use of antithyroid medication and/or beta blockers, or natural agents such as bugleweed, motherwort, and L-carnitine. While I'm all for using the natural agents, if someone has a very high resting heart rate then it might be wise to take the medication while at the same time trying to address the underlying cause of the condition. So taking a natural treatment approach shouldn't increase the risk if one takes the proper precautions.

Question #16: Can Someone Who Has Already Received Radioactive Iodine Treatment Restore Their Thyroid Health?

The goal here isn't to offer false hope to people who have already received radioactive iodine treatment. So let me begin by stating that for someone who has already received RAI, it will be much more difficult to restore their health when compared to someone who hasn't received this treatment procedure. On the other hand, some people who have received RAI can restore their thyroid health. This doesn't mean that natural treatment methods will completely reverse the damage caused by the radioactive iodine, but sometimes it can get the thyroid gland to a point where it will produce a sufficient amount of thyroid hormone on its own so that the person doesn't need to take synthetic or natural thyroid hormone on a permanent basis.

Of course there is a decent chance that someone who has received radioactive iodine won't have their thyroid health restored back to normal, and may need to take thyroid hormone continuously. But as I have mentioned many times in this book, radioactive iodine won't do anything to address the cause of hyperthyroidism and Graves' disease. So even if it's not possible to get the thyroid gland to produce a sufficient amount of thyroid hormone on its own, most of these people still can benefit from natural treatment methods in order to restore the health of other areas which may be compromised (adrenal glands, immune system, digestive system, etc.).

Question #17: Do You Work With New Patients?

As of writing this book I do accept a limited number of new patients each month. For more information, visit the website workwithdreric.com.

Question #18: Can Poor Oral Health Cause A Thyroid Condition?

Most of us don't think about the potential impact that poor oral health can have on our entire body. The truth is that there are numerous problems with the teeth and gums which can potentially lead to chronic health conditions. I discussed mercury fillings earlier in this book, as this can have a negative impact on one's health. Gingivitis is a source of inflammation that probably won't trigger an autoimmune response, but then again, any inflammation in the body can cause problems. There is also some evidence that root canals can lead to numerous health issues, as the fear is that a root canal can eventually lead to an infection (even after they sterilize the canal), and this in turn can potentially lead to certain health conditions. And since every tooth correlates with a specific body meridian, having a root canal on a tooth that correlates with the thyroid gland might have a negative impact on thyroid health. What I recommend is for everyone to consider seeing a biological dentist, who will take a more natural approach to dental health. You can find a biological dentist through the International Academy of Oral Medicine and Toxicology (IAOMT). Their website is www.IAOMT.org.

Question #19: Can People With Subacute Thyroiditis Benefit From Taking A Natural Treatment Approach?

Subacute thyroiditis is a condition which involves inflammation of the thyroid gland, and it usually is caused by a virus. Both the radioactive iodine uptake test and thyroid stimulating immunoglobulins will usually be negative. With subacute thyroiditis, hyperthyroidism will usually last for about 2 to 3 months, and frequently is followed by a period of hypothyroidism, which might also be temporary, but in some cases may be permanent. Natural treatment methods may help someone with thyroiditis, although this condition may resolve on its own without the person taking a natural treatment approach. However, even if the state of hyperthyroidism is temporary, it still is important to manage the hyperthyroid symptoms through medication, or through herbs such as bugleweed and/or motherwort.

Question #20: What Can Be Done For Hair Loss Caused By Hyperthyroidism?

Many people with hyperthyroidism experience hair loss, and while this might not be the most concerning symptom someone with this condition has, it is still very distressing for many people. This is especially true since hyperthyroidism is more common in women, and over the years I have worked with many women with hyperthyroidism who were stressed out the most over their hair loss.

The good news is that in most cases the person's hair loss will stop and grow back. Of course it can take time for this to happen, and one also needs to keep in mind that there can be other causes of hair loss, including nutrient deficiencies and sex hormone imbalances. It's also worth mentioning that while taking antithyroid medication can sometimes help with hair loss, other times it will worsen it. Either way, the goal should still be to do things to address the underlying cause of the hyperthyroid condition.

Question #21: Can Hyperthyroidism Cause Osteoporosis?

I briefly mentioned this in Chapter 20, as unmanaged hyperthyroidism can cause a decrease in bone density, and in some cases can cause osteoporosis. This is yet another reason why you want to take hyperthyroidism seriously, and even if you don't experience any cardiovascular symptoms (i.e. elevated pulse rate, heart palpitations), elevated thyroid hormones can decrease bone density. The good news is that you can reverse osteopenia, and even osteoporosis, although it of course is best to try to prevent it from developing in the first place.

Balancing the thyroid hormones is of course important, and having healthy estrogen levels is also essential. Also important is having healthy vitamin D levels, and other nutrients are of course important for optimal bone health as well, including calcium, magnesium, vitamin K2, and boron. Regular exercise can also be beneficial, especially weight bearing exercise. For more information please check out my interview with Kevin Ellis on my podcast, which you can listen to by visiting savemythyroid.com/58.

Question #22: Are There Concerns with Oxalates and Vegetable Consumption?

I have a few blog posts and podcast episodes related to oxalates, which are small molecules that have the ability to form crystals, which in turn can deposit in different areas of the body, including the thyroid gland. What's scary is that some of the foods higher in oxalates are allowed on many diets considered to be healthy, including Paleo and AIP. These include spinach, Swiss chard, blackberries, raspberries, and sweet potatoes.

I'm sure some people who are familiar with oxalates cringed when I mentioned that I drink smoothies on a daily basis. But I will say that the smoothie I make is probably lower in oxalates than the "average" smoothie, as I include lower oxalate green leafy vegetables such as lettuces (romaine, green leaf, red leaf), arugula, and collard greens. While I do add some blackberries and raspberries at times, I also add berries lower in oxalates such as blueberries and cranberries.

For more information on oxalates you can check out my blog posts and/or podcast episodes. And my book the Hyperthyroid Healing Diet, which will be released the first quarter of 2024, will also have a chapter dedicated to oxalates.

Question #23: What Do You Think About Utilizing Other Alternative Treatment Methods With Regards To Treating Hyperthyroid Conditions?

1. **Chiropractic.** Although some chiropractors like myself help people with conditions such as hyperthyroidism and Graves' disease, chiropractic care itself won't provide a cure for this condition. This doesn't mean that chiropractic care can't benefit people with hyperthyroidism.

While most people perceive chiropractors as being neck and back pain doctors, chiropractic is more than just helping people get relief from their pain. I'm not going to get into detail about chiropractic, but chiropractors deal with subluxations, which essentially are misalignments that affect the nervous system. As you probably know, the nerves communicate with every organ, tissue, and cell in the body. And so while a subluxation can cause pain, it can definitely lead to more serious health issues.

For example, if someone has a subluxation affecting the nerves which supply the thyroid gland, then it's possible this can affect one's thyroid health. Can it lead to a hyperthyroid condition? I honestly don't know, but if I had such a subluxation I know that I would want to have it corrected. Similarly, subluxations can affect any other gland or organ in the body. Having one or more subluxations can also affect the immune system as well, which obviously is very important in people with Graves' disease. So while chiropractic care itself isn't required to restore the health of most people with hyperthyroidism, having one or more subluxations can potentially affect someone's recovery, and from an overall health perspective, many people with hyperthyroidism can benefit from chiropractic care.

2. **Acupuncture.** Just as is the case with chiropractic, many people can benefit from acupuncture. But receiving acupuncture alone usually won't restore the health of someone who has hyperthyroidism. On the other hand, combining acupuncture with changes in lifestyle factors, along with certain supplements and/or herbs will be more effective. So both chiropractic care and acupuncture can benefit the health of people with hyperthyroid conditions, and remove some interferences which can potentially prevent someone from restoring their health. But just receiving chiropractic care or acupuncture alone usually won't be sufficient to restore one's health.

3. Homeopathy. I personally don't know anyone with hyperthyroidism who has restored their health by solely using homeopathic remedies, but this doesn't mean that homeopathy can't be beneficial. I would definitely give homeopathy a try before receiving radioactive iodine or thyroid surgery. If seeking a healthcare professional who uses homeopathy I would try to work with someone who focuses on thyroid and autoimmune thyroid conditions.

When it comes down to it, I do think there are different ways of accomplishing the same thing. In other words, different natural healthcare practitioners will have different recommendations, and when it comes to avoiding radioactive iodine treatment and preserving the health of your thyroid gland, I think these alternative treatment methods can be beneficial, although I wouldn't expect any of these alone to restore your thyroid and immune health.

Thank you for reading my book!

I really appreciate all of your feedback and
I love hearing what you have to say.

I need your input to make the next version of
this book and my future books better.

Please take two minutes now to leave a helpful review on
Amazon letting me know what you thought of the book.

You can do so by visiting savemythyroid.com/review

Also, I'd love to read your review, and so after you leave it
please let me know by sending an email to
info@naturalendocrinesolutions.com

Want to work with my team and I?

If you have hyperthyroidism and want to do everything you can to save your thyroid, then there are a few factors that can prevent someone from restoring their health:

1. Overlooking the fundamentals
2. Lack of full commitment
3. Lack of accountability
4. Not working with a practitioner who has experience with hyperthyroidism

By reading this book you should have a good grasp of the foundations when it comes to restoring your health, although you can also check out my free Foundations of Overcoming Hyperthyroidism Online Course at savemythyroid.com/foundations. Of course only you can make the commitment to do what is necessary to save your thyroid, but if you want more guidance and accountability and would like to learn what it's like to work with my team and I visit workwithdreric.com.

About The Author

DR. ERIC OSANSKY is a licensed chiropractor with a masters degree in nutrition, and is also an Institute for Functional Medicine Certified Practitioner (IFMCP). Dr. Eric was diagnosed with Graves' disease in 2008, and restored his health through natural treatment methods. Dr. Osansky graduated summa cum laude from Life Chiropractic College in March of 1999, and like most other chiropractors he initially focused on musculoskeletal conditions, and did so for 7 1/2 years. But after restoring his health he began to exclusively see people with thyroid and autoimmune thyroid conditions, and approximately 85% of his patient base consists of those with hyperthyroidism.

In addition to his extensive background in nutrition and functional medicine he has obtained hundreds of hours of post-graduate training in neuroendocrinology, immunology, biotransformation and detoxification, and phytotherapy. He has also received a certificate of practical herbal therapy from the Australian College of Phytotherapy.

While Dr. Osansky feels that most people with hyperthyroidism should give natural treatment methods a try, he does realize that there is a time and place for conventional medical treatment such as antithyroid medication, and even thyroid surgery in certain situations. And while he of course wants to help everyone with hyperthyroidism, Dr. Osansky won't hesitate to refer someone out if he feels as if they are not a good candidate for a natural treatment approach.

As of writing this book Dr. Osansky does accept a limited number of new patients each month for people with thyroid and autoimmune thyroid conditions looking to restore their health naturally. Those who are interested in working with Dr. Eric should visit workwithdreric.com.

Dr. Osansky lives in Matthews, NC, with his wife Cindy, and his two teenage daughters, Marissa and Jaylee.

Index

A

Acid-Stopping medication 98
Acupuncture 360
Addison's disease 64, 75
Adrenal fatigue 73, 81
Adrenal glands 6, 15, 31, 36, 38, 42, 43,
   57, 71, 72, 73, 74, 75, 76, 77, 78, 81,
   86, 87, 144, 145, 202, 217, 226, 308,
   313, 353, 356
Adrenal Stress Index Test 57
Adrenal testing 76, 203, 298
Air fresheners 165, 168
Alcohol 353
Alpha lipoic acid 146, 178, 258
Aluminum 172, 173, 180
Antibodies 11, 16, 22, 30, 31, 32, 33,
   56, 69, 79, 100, 103, 105, 120, 136,
   184, 200, 201, 202, 203, 205, 207,
   208, 216, 234, 247, 254, 257, 263,
   264, 266, 274, 298, 307, 352
Antithyroid drugs 1, 4, 13, 14, 17, 23,
   36, 43, 45, 46, 49, 50, 51, 53, 65, 70,
   136, 202, 206, 209, 211, 213, 215,
   216, 222, 223, 224, 225, 226, 227,
   228, 229, 231, 232, 233, 234, 235,
   237, 238, 243, 267, 268, 269, 278,
   280, 297, 329, 337, 338, 348
Arsenic 172, 174, 180
Asthma 168
Atrial Fibrillation 233
Autoimmune Epidemic 39, 72, 163,
   179, 194

B

Ballantyne, Dr. Sarah 118, 127
Banik, Dr. Rani 265
Berberine 187, 258, 259
Beta blocker 23, 64, 65, 134, 136, 202,
   228, 232, 233, 238, 350
Betaine HCL 93, 95, 107, 141, 142
Biofeedback 320
Blood sugar levels 114, 116, 353
Blood tests 5, 11, 12, 22, 24, 35, 55, 56,
   60, 61, 112, 131, 199, 200, 202, 210,
   231, 291, 292, 306, 317, 328
Bone density 92, 234, 350, 351, 358
Brazil nuts 136
Breastfeeding 17, 206, 208, 267, 268,
   270, 271, 272, 273, 275, 276
Broccoli 96, 123, 146, 274
Brownstein, Dr. David 161
Brussels sprouts 126
Bugleweed 17, 54, 127, 131, 134, 135,
   136, 145, 149, 150, 211, 216, 233,
   234, 235, 236, 238, 269, 271, 272,
   273, 278, 279, 280, 291, 292, 308,
   309, 310, 316, 339, 344, 349, 350,
   355, 357
B vitamins 142, 154

C

Cadmium 172, 174, 180
Candida overgrowth 101, 185
Caprylic Acid 188
Castor oil packs 240, 250, 251
Cat's Claw 188, 191

Cauliflower 146, 319
Celiac Disease 64, 79, 80, 113, 319
Childbearing age 167, 213
Chiropractic 2, 4, 21, 25, 47, 58, 85, 104, 298, 352, 359, 360
Cholestyramine 18, 211, 217, 310, 311, 316, 350
Cigarette smoking 171
Coffee enemas 179
Colloidal Silver 189
Colon Hydrotherapy 179, 305
Comprehensive stool panel 57, 61, 89, 90, 131, 185, 298, 305, 350
Constipation 95, 96, 111, 137, 305
Conventional medical treatment 4, 8, 9, 13, 14, 15, 32, 36, 45, 48, 49, 106, 206, 254, 255, 256, 262, 263, 266, 277, 279, 281, 289, 290, 316, 340, 365
Copper deficiency 144
Copper toxicity 144, 145
CoQ10 142, 143, 228
Corticosteroids 73, 254, 256, 260, 262, 263, 264
Cortisol levels 6, 57, 72, 73, 76, 77, 81, 86, 148, 304, 305
Crinnion, Dr. Walter 40, 170
Cyrex Labs 79, 99, 100, 102, 103, 105, 109
Cytomegalovirus 183, 186, 191

D
Dairy 93, 99, 101, 104, 106, 113, 114, 115, 119, 126, 146, 165, 257, 303, 318, 319, 338
Danish population 160
Dentistry model 300
Detoxification program 22, 122, 324
DHEA 57, 77, 78, 81, 86, 305
Digestion 15, 89, 93, 94, 95, 96
Digestive enzymes 91, 93, 95, 107, 141, 150, 322
Distilled water 125
Dried urine testing 80, 81, 239

E
Eggs 119, 120, 124, 354
Electrolytes 179, 323
Eleuthero 147
Elimination diet 15, 104, 118, 119, 120, 122, 129
Ellis, Kevin 358
Endocrinologist 1, 2, 22, 23, 35, 36, 53, 56, 63, 64, 70, 74, 75, 202, 210, 211, 218, 221, 223, 231, 232, 235, 237, 238, 239, 245, 251, 283, 297, 298, 309, 311, 330, 335, 337, 349, 350
Environmental toxins xv, 16, 163, 175
Epigenetics 195
Epstein-Barr Virus 182
Estrogen 42, 80, 117, 147, 155, 157, 158, 165, 166, 169, 180, 239, 240, 241, 247, 248, 250, 283, 284, 285, 286, 287, 289, 290, 348, 354, 358
Estrogen dominance 285
Estrogen metabolism 80, 155, 157, 158, 169, 239, 240, 241, 247, 248, 250, 283, 284, 285, 286, 287, 289, 290, 348
Exercise 84, 351
Exophthalmos 254, 255

F
Fiber 95, 96, 97, 107, 321
Fine Needle Aspiration 242
Fish oils 131, 137, 149, 150, 322
Food allergies 324
Food diary 122
Food sensitivities 74, 78, 102, 104, 107, 118, 119, 120, 129
Free T3 200
Free T4 22, 311

G
Gaining weight (with hyperthyroidism) 19, 354
Gamma-linolenic acid 144
Garlic 188, 191

Gastrointestinal tract 74, 100, 108, 109, 188, 259

Genetics 16, 42, 193, 201

GI-MAP 184

Gliadin AB 79

Glutathione 146, 178, 179, 258, 286

Gluten 79, 80, 93, 99, 101, 104, 113, 114, 115, 116, 126, 257, 303, 304, 318, 319, 338, 347, 348

Goiter 18, 19, 247, 283, 284, 287, 289, 348

Goitrogens 129, 284

Goldenseal 187, 191, 259

Grains 94, 114, 115, 116, 119, 121, 129

Graves Disease 19, 30, 200, 345

Graves' ophthalmopathy 254, 257, 258, 262, 263, 266

Gut microbiome 31, 37, 38, 42, 43, 44, 92, 93, 95, 96, 97, 101, 106, 108, 109, 187, 190, 217, 227, 241, 242, 257, 259, 264, 286, 305

H

Hair loss 19, 357

Hair Mineral Analysis 58, 131, 172, 203

Hashimoto's Thyroiditis 4, 25, 26, 32, 64, 81, 153, 183, 200, 201, 203, 285, 306, 329, 332, 343, 352

HeartMath 82, 320

Heavy Metals 16, 40, 68, 157, 170, 172, 175

Helicobacter Pylori 39, 41, 106, 183, 184, 186, 188, 189, 191

Hepatitis C 41, 183, 184, 186, 191

Herbs 16, 107, 131, 133, 142, 147, 149, 187, 257, 271

High cortisol 57, 72, 76, 78, 148, 354

High energy levels 86

Homeopathy 361

Hyperthyroid diet xv, 15, 111

Hyperthyroid healing community 345

Hyperthyroid healing diet 37, 66, 111, 114, 123, 345, 359

Hyperthyroidism 12, 14, 15, 16, 19, 23, 29, 37, 43, 71, 126, 131, 142, 151, 158, 160, 208, 275, 299, 344, 345, 347, 348, 350, 351, 354, 357, 358, 364

Hypothalamic-pituitary-adrenal (HPA) axis 147

Hypothyroidism 4, 5, 24, 26, 27, 35, 127, 143, 150, 158, 171, 210, 233, 244, 268, 271, 285, 313, 315, 329, 352, 353, 357

I

Immune system (compromised, overactive, weak, etc.) 15, 30, 31, 32, 33, 36, 39, 40, 41, 42, 57, 63, 64, 65, 66, 67, 68, 69, 70, 72, 73, 74, 78, 100, 108, 109, 139, 140, 164, 166, 171, 178, 181, 182, 187, 190, 196, 200, 201, 202, 203, 217, 226, 255, 256, 259, 261, 264, 265, 272, 300, 306, 307, 340, 356, 360

Infrared sauna 179, 305, 324

Insomnia 135, 136, 137

Institute for Functional Medicine 25, 365

Insulin resistance 67, 116, 117, 126, 157, 187, 239, 241, 242, 248, 250, 258, 287, 289, 290, 348, 354

International Academy of Oral Medicine and Toxicology 173, 178, 357

Intestinal permeability 38, 43, 60, 67, 69, 78, 91, 101, 103, 108, 109, 179

Iodine 1, 2, 5, 7, 13, 16, 22, 23, 25, 26, 30, 32, 35, 36, 43, 45, 50, 56, 61, 63, 64, 145, 149, 151, 152, 153, 154, 155, 156, 157, 158, 159, 160, 161, 162, 202, 204, 205, 206, 207, 208, 209, 210, 211, 212, 213, 214, 215, 216, 217, 218, 219, 220, 221, 222, 223, 224, 225, 226, 236, 242, 243, 244, 245, 249, 250, 251, 255, 256, 263, 264, 268, 278, 279, 284, 285, 287, 288, 289, 290, 292, 297, 308, 309, 311, 312, 313, 314, 315, 316, 333,

337, 338, 339, 340, 341, 342, 348,
349, 350, 351, 355, 356, 357, 361
Iron 3, 144, 175, 270

K

Kale 146, 274
Kidney 145, 174, 299

L

Lactation 17, 267, 271, 273
L-Carnitine 135
Lead 175
Leaky gut 38, 43, 60, 67, 91, 99, 100,
101, 102, 103, 104, 105, 106, 108,
109, 227, 308, 353
Lectins 121
Lee, Dr. John R. 166
Lemon Balm 131, 135, 136, 150, 273
L-glutamine 91, 107, 109
Lifestyle factors 59, 61, 92, 128, 164,
165, 180, 194, 195, 196, 300, 318,
325, 339, 360
Lithium 145
Liver enzymes 226
Low cortisol 57, 73, 76
Low dose naltrexone (LDN) 18, 217,
253, 261, 306, 316, 350
Lyme disease 41, 56, 184, 185, 186,
189, 190

M

Magnesium 137, 322
Maintaining your health 190
Mastic Gum 191
Mazza, Dr. Angela 249
Mediator release testing 105, 117, 120,
129
Mercury 68, 172, 174, 180, 356
Methimazole 13, 23, 53, 64, 101, 109,
132, 149, 209, 211, 216, 223, 225,
226, 227, 235, 236, 264, 268, 278,
283, 308, 309, 310, 311, 316, 349, 350
Methylation 142, 286, 322

Moore, Elaine 12, 200, 266
Motherwort 17, 54, 127, 131, 134, 135,
136, 150, 233, 234, 235, 236, 238,
269, 273, 278, 291, 292, 339, 355,
357
Multinodular Goiter 18, 247, 283, 284,
287, 289
Muscle mass 115, 351

N

N-acetyl-cysteine 146
Nakazawa, Donna Jackson 72, 163, 164,
194
Natural Endocrine solutions 19, 344
Natural thyroid health xvi, 19
Nightshades 94, 115, 118, 119, 120,
129, 257
Nutritional deficiencies 38, 39, 43, 67,
101, 121, 164, 180
Nutritional supplements 16, 131, 133,
270, 321

O

Olive leaf 189, 191
Omega 3 Fatty Acids 258
Optimal health (receiving) 108, 197,
247, 299, 300, 301, 305, 323, 337, 339
Optimal results (receiving) 294, 295,
303, 316, 328, 334, 341, 353
Oral health 356
Oregano oil 187, 191
Organic 40, 58, 106, 113, 121, 123,
125, 128, 165, 169, 170, 171, 174,
185, 338, 352, 354
Osteoporosis 358
Oxalates 359

P

Pau D' Arco 188, 191
Peaches 126
Pesticides 165
Pharmaceutical companies 13, 46
Picky eaters 352

Pituitary gland 72
Prebiotics 93, 107, 109, 321
Pregnancy 127, 158, 268, 269, 270, 271, 272, 273, 274, 275
Probiotics 107, 140, 188, 191
Progesterone 78, 80, 286
Propranolol 311
Propylthiouracil (PTU) 13, 101, 215, 224
Pulse rate 21, 22, 24, 54, 134, 224, 233, 238, 350, 351, 358
Purified water 123, 125, 176, 323, 338

Q
Quercetin 189, 191, 259

R
Radioactive Iodine (receiving treatment after, getting over the anger, risks, precautions) 16, 204, 205, 208, 209, 215, 218, 219, 220, 255, 268, 312, 344, 348, 355, 371
Radioactive Iodine Uptake test 16, 22, 30, 204, 205, 206, 207, 208, 357
Radiofrequency ablation 17, 240, 243, 244, 251, 252, 289, 290, 314, 349
Recipe books 127
Refined foods 54, 59, 77, 99, 101, 112, 113, 114, 121, 123, 129, 174, 318, 319, 325, 338
Relapse 55, 59, 60, 113, 184, 196, 197, 198, 224, 225, 226, 229, 300, 301, 318, 320
Remission 5, 13, 17, 23, 36, 39, 53, 54, 55, 56, 58, 60, 61, 114, 197, 198, 202, 211, 216, 223, 225, 226, 229, 297, 315, 324, 331, 347
Resistance exercise 351
Resveratrol 147, 259
Reverse osmosis 125

S
Save My Thyroid Quiz 345
Secretory IgA 57, 73, 74, 78, 79, 103

Selenium 69, 136, 137, 146, 150, 154, 156, 162, 178, 257, 270
Self-treat 23, 24, 43, 272, 280, 292, 293, 294, 295, 296, 334, 341
Sex hormones 80, 308, 340, 354, 355
Shomon, Mary J. 12
Siberian Ginseng 147
Silver fillings 177
Sleep deprivation 67
Soy 93, 114, 115, 126, 257, 338, 354
Spinach 126
Spinal Subluxations 4, 298
Statins 49, 143
Stealth infections 185
Strawberries 126
Stress 6, 15, 37, 38, 39, 40, 43, 44, 54, 59, 66, 67, 68, 70, 71, 72, 73, 74, 75, 76, 77, 78, 81, 82, 83, 84, 85, 86, 87, 92, 96, 97, 101, 109, 114, 128, 142, 145, 146, 147, 150, 153, 154, 156, 169, 178, 181, 187, 247, 256, 258, 272, 275, 285, 293, 299, 301, 304, 313, 317, 318, 320, 323, 324, 325, 339
Stress management 15, 66, 83, 85, 87, 256, 320, 323, 324, 339
Subacute thyroiditis 357
Subclinical Hyperthyroidism 19, 275, 350
Subluxation 299, 360
Symptom management 3, 23, 134, 135, 236, 262, 269, 280, 353
Symptoms (of hyperthyroidism) 23, 53, 56, 58, 131, 134, 135, 145, 209, 210, 212, 213, 220, 223, 224, 227, 229, 233, 234, 235, 238, 247, 278, 279, 280, 294, 312, 314, 315, 317, 349, 355, 357

T
TGI 200
Th1 Pathway 203, 204
Th2 pathway 203, 204
Thyroglobulin antibodies 32, 201

Thyroid antibodies 11, 16, 22, 30, 32, 56, 69, 136, 200, 201, 202, 203, 205, 207, 208, 216, 247, 257, 263, 274, 298, 307
Thyroid biopsy 246
Thyroid calming bundle 132
Thyroid cancer 217
Thyroidectomy 213, 218, 244, 264, 283, 287, 288, 289, 290, 312, 313, 314, 315, 340
Thyroid eye disease 17, 47, 147, 187, 207, 214, 215, 253, 254, 255, 257, 258, 259, 260, 264, 265, 266
Thyroid eye disease bundle 259
Thyroid health resources 19
Thyroid inhibition 160
Thyroiditis 4, 25, 26, 32, 64, 81, 153, 154, 183, 200, 201, 203, 205, 285, 306, 329, 332, 343, 352, 357
Thyroid nodules (Malignant, Physical Obstruction) 17, 80, 155, 157, 158, 204, 206, 208, 239, 240, 241, 242, 243, 244, 245, 246, 248, 249, 250, 251, 252, 284, 285, 286, 288, 290, 349
Thyroid peroxidase antibodies 201
Thyroid stimulating immunoglobulins 24, 89, 90, 199, 201, 203, 204, 205, 206, 208, 210, 254, 257, 287, 313, 357
Thyroid storm (Managing The Symptoms, Preventing, Triggers) 17, 135, 234, 277, 278, 279, 280, 281
Thyrotoxicosis 215, 274
Toxic multinodular goiter 18, 25, 30, 151, 169, 228, 229, 247, 283, 284, 286, 287, 288, 289, 290
Triad of autoimmunity 91
TSH 22, 24, 31, 32, 33, 35, 53, 135, 136, 200, 203, 210, 214, 231, 234, 236, 237, 260, 263, 264, 269, 274, 275, 284, 285, 298, 313, 350

TSH receptor antibodies 31, 32, 33, 234, 264, 274
Turmeric 147, 259
Turnips 126

U
Ultrasonography 240, 245
Unfermented Soy 126

V
Vegetarian 94, 115, 121, 138, 353, 354
vitamin C 144, 154, 258
vitamin D 84, 138, 139, 140, 150, 258, 358
Vitt, Carrie 251
Volatile Organic Compounds (VOCs) 40, 170

W
Water 103, 106, 123, 125, 170, 173, 174, 175, 176, 323, 338
Weight gain 226, 354
Weight loss 22
Wentz, Dr. Izabella 81
Whole foods 98, 99, 112, 121, 128, 137, 303, 319, 325, 338
Wormwood 189, 191

X
Xenoestrogens 165, 166, 167, 180
Xenohormones 16, 40, 165, 166, 167

Y
Yersinia enterocolitica 41, 69, 183, 184, 191

Z
Zinc 101, 108, 109

Printed in the USA
CPSIA information can be obtained
at www.ICGtesting.com
LVHW020158030424
776277LV00007B/276